8 Weeks to SEAL**FIT**

A NAVY SEAL'S

GUIDE TO

UNCONVENTIONAL

TRAINING FOR

PHYSICAL AND

MENTAL

TOUGHNESS

8 Weeks to SEALFIT

MARK DIVINE

ST. MARTIN'S GRIFFIN NEW YORK

ALSO BY MARK DIVINE

Unbeatable Mind

The Way of the SEAL

8 WEEKS TO SEALFIT. Copyright © 2014 by Mark Divine. Foreword copyright © 2014 by Joe Stumpf. All rights reserved. Printed in the United States of America. For information, address St. Martin's Press, 175 Fifth Avenue, New York, N.Y. 10010.

Book designed by Richard Oriolo

www.stmartins.com

Library of Congress Cataloging-in-Publication Data

Divine, Mark.
   8 weeks to SEALFIT : a Navy SEAL's guide to unconventional training for physical and mental toughness / Mark Divine.
      pp. cm.
   ISBN 978-1-250-04054-1 (paperback)
   ISBN 978-1-4668-3589-4 (e-book)
1. Divine, Mark. 2. Exercise. 3. Physical fitness. 4. United States. Navy. SEALs—Physical training.
5. United States. Navy. SEALs—Anecdotes. I. Title. II. Title: Eight weeks to SEALFIT, a Navy SEAL's guide to unconventional training for physical and mental toughness. III. Title: Navy SEAL's guide to unconventional training for physical and mental toughness.
   GV481.D587 2014
   613.7—dc23

                                                                                2013032035

St. Martin's Griffin books may be purchased for educational, business, or promotional use. For information on bulk purchases, please contact Macmillan Corporate and Premium Sales Department at 1-800-221-7945, extension 5442, or write specialmarkets@macmillan.com.

FIRST EDITION: April 2014

10 9 8 7 6 5 4 3 2 1

CONTENTS

ACKNOWLEDGMENTS

NOTHING WORTHY IS ACCOMPLISHED ALONE. My philosophy for life and physical fitness has been forged through nearly 25 years of training, trial, and error. I've been influenced by many mentors over the years, many of whom have little idea of the impact they've had on me.

I'm heavily indebted to Mr. Kaicho Tadashi Nakamura. He was my teacher for Seido Karate—a traditional martial art—during the late 1980s, when I earned my first black belt. Kaicho taught me many of the mental toughness principles that helped me sail through BUD/S and that are included in SEALFIT.

My yoga mentor, Tim Miller, is another gem. I train in Ashtanga Yoga with Tim in my hometown of Encinitas, California. Tim is the first American yoga instructor certified by Sri K. Pattabhi Jois, the founder of modern Ashtanga Yoga. The roots of Ashtanga Yoga are over 4,000 years old and considered a "fast track" for the eight limbs of yoga for athletes and warriors. Tim's trainings are often 2 hours in length. They include a breath control *pranayama* session that spans 50 minutes, which often leaves me gasping. Tim teaches me humility, the value of practicing daily, and the importance of teaching weekly. Anything else would remove the teacher too far from leading from the front and experiencing firsthand what you're asking your trainees to experience. I've personally adopted this principle and I like to say that I eat my own dog food at SEALFIT. I'd like to thank Kaicho and Tim, as well as their teachers, for their wonderful examples of warrior mastery.

Tom Brown, from the Tracker School, and Shannon Phelps, of Saito Ninjutusu, have had a significant influence on my thinking and development. I'm grateful to both, as well as to their teachers.

I'm grateful to my SEALFIT coaches—Chriss Smith, Dan Cerrillo, Brad McLeod, Lance Cummings, Charlie Moser, Shane Hiatt, Chris Haskell, Sean Lake, Dan Miller, Derek Price, and the late Glen Doherty—for their loyalty, incredible coaching skills, and humor. I'm grateful to my interns—especially Joe L.—for being my gofers and training guinea pigs.

I owe a debt of gratitude to CrossFit, Inc., and Coach Greg Glassman for the influence that CrossFit has had on my own training and SEALFIT methods.

I'm grateful to my Olympic lifting coach, Mike Burgener, for his training and inspiration. I'm also grateful to his son, Beau, and Rob Shaul of Military Athlete for their support and hours of training and lessons.

Though we haven't met yet, I'm grateful to Ken Wilber for his groundbreaking work in Integral Theory. When I stumbled upon Ken's writing, I immediately recognized that we were kindred spirits and that SEALFIT was an "Integral Warrior Development" program. I'm thankful that Ken gave me the words to define, research, and validate the program. I'm also grateful to Michael Ostrolenk for his integral contributions to SEALFIT, as well as the Unbeatable Mind Academy.

I have many great friends and supporters who have made my life an amazing journey. I'd like to thank Rob Ord, who stuck with me after the U.S. Tactical contract loss and helped me launch US CrossFit and the Kokoro Camp. I'd like to also thank Brandon Webb of SOFREP—the author of *The Red Circle*—who helped me get a book deal in two weeks with a very rough manuscript.

I'm grateful to my SEALFIT staff, especially Rich Vernetti, Cindy Chapman, Catherine Chapman, Melanie Sliwka, and my writing coach, Peter Nevland, of the Wizard Academy. Without Peter this would be a very different book.

I'm grateful beyond words for all my teammates who have sacrificed for this country—especially my friend and SEALFIT coach Glen Doherty.

I'm eternally grateful to my mom, who introduced me to the world of sports, and to my dad, who taught me the value of hard work and doing things right.

And to my wife, Sandy, who has supported my crazy adventures with a smile (most of the time) and always with grace. Also my son, Devon, who keeps me laughing and honest.

Hooyah, Team!

MY NAME IS JOE STUMPF. In the world of business, I own one of the largest business and life coaching companies in the country. I am privileged to work with some of the most successful entrepreneurs and businesspeople every day. I have invested hundreds of hours and tens of thousands of dollars on personal development and spiritual awareness coaching programs and workshops throughout the last 20 years.

One of my most significant accomplishments up to this point in my life is, at age 54, I completed the civilian version of the Navy SEAL Hell Week—Mark Divine's Kokoro Camp. Because of my unique point of view and exposure to the world's best coaches—plus training daily at Mark's SEALFIT/US Crossfit center in Encinitas—I'm the perfect person to share with you what an extraordinary opportunity you have in your hands right now with the book *8 Weeks to SEALFIT*.

I met Mark at a pivotal turning point of my life. Having achieved business success and enjoying great relationships with family and friends, I was reexamining my bigger purpose in life for the next 50 years, and I wanted to finish strong. I had seen far too many men, including my father, finish life getting weaker emotionally, mentally, spiritually, and physically, and I knew that if I didn't make it my primary purpose to get stronger as I grew older, I could easily slip down that path, too.

In my business coaching program, we guide people in business through the four phases of growth. Survival to Stability, Stability to Success, and Success to Significance. In my experience, I have witnessed thousands of men and women go through these stages, and yet the stage from Success to Significance seems to be reserved for only the few that dare to fully reinvent themselves after they have achieved worldly success. Making money and accumulating power and prestige is a matter of drive, determination, smart strategic direction, and being at the right place at the right time—taking advantage of the opportunities as they present themselves. The more elusive stage of growth is Significance, because it seems to invite us into a way of being that requires a completely different awareness. When we get to that place and are ready to make the shift, we discover what got us here won't get us there. This is the place I found myself in early 2010. I was having a conversation with Mark and I asked him if he thought I had what it took to get through Kokoro. He said, "Joe, only you would know!" I asked him what would be the biggest benefit I would receive if I choose to do what was necessary to achieve that goal. He said, "Joe, within you is a voice that is yet to be born; it is the voice of your most authentic self. You can continue through life constantly upgrading what you have already mastered or you can give rise to a version of yourself that is the most powerful loving self. To do that you must choose to follow the path of the warrior—a path few men dare to travel. But when you do, you will meet yourself for the very first time."

The right words from the right person at the right time can change your destiny. Mark's words spoke to my soul, and that voice within—the one only you could hear if you were willing to. I started training with Mark and his SEALFIT team every Monday, Wednesday, and Friday. (You can check out his workouts at SEALFIT'S Web site, www.sealfit.com.) The workouts are rough and long, and they require strength, stamina, and endurance. But most of all, they require a commitment to wholeheartedness. Mark watched over me as my body got destroyed, but my mind and spirit toughened. He said, "Joe, just show up no matter what. Once you get here, everything will work itself out." In AA, they say bring the body and the mind will follow. I trusted Mark and I showed up for almost a year and he was right. I was now in the best physical and mental condition of my life. I enrolled in his 3-week academy and moved into the SEALFIT facility with four other boys all half my age. We trained in Mark's Five Mountains of SEALFIT approach 10 hours a day, 7 days a week, with him and his team of extraordinary leaders. During this time, I discovered how little I really needed in the material world. The essence of life was found in teamwork, discipline, and love for my fellow man. I learned what it meant to drop the ego and show up every minute fully present. I was there and he fully prepared me to discover if I had the *secret sauce*—the ingredient that is in all of us if we choose to live a life of significance.

I made it through the 50-hour Kokoro Camp, and Mark presented me with the Fire in the Gut Award for my courage to overcome insurmountable obstacles. I credit this achievement to his brilliant mentorship.

With the book, *8 Weeks to SEALFIT,* you have in your hands the exact blueprint I followed to lead my life in the direction of significance. Of course you will get into the best condition of your life, but something even more magical is available if you follow his teaching completely. You may discover that voice within that wants to finish strong, wants to express its most authentic part of you, and to make a contribution to the world.

What I want for you is the experience of having Mark Divine mentor you, like Obi-Wan Kenobi mentored Luke Skywalker, so that you too can discover your true significance.

—JOE STUMPF
Author of *Willing Warrior*
Cardiff-by-the-Sea, California

WHEN I ATTENDED KOKORO CAMP, SEALFIT's grueling 50-hour crucible experience in 2011, I was struck by how important mental preparation is to success. Prior to the camp, I had heard the oft-repeated phrase that crucible experiences are 80 percent mental and 20 percent physical. It isn't until sleep deprivation and exhaustion take hold, however, that a person truly understands the accuracy of that statement. The camp also made me realize how I, and many others in my class, were lacking from a physical standpoint. We had guys who could run all day but struggled under the weight of a rucksack, and others who were strong as an ox but lacked endurance. These imbalances grew more pronounced as the weekend progressed and fatigue set in. When I finished the camp and had an opportunity to reflect on my experience I realized that success in Kokoro, and in life for that matter, is largely dependent upon one thing: balance.

SEALFIT is the epitome of balance. It involves making an honest assessment of yourself, determining your weaknesses, and committing yourself to personal improvement every day. Over time an individual who does this becomes balanced across all areas. Physically, they have strength and endurance, power and flexibility. Mentally, they have the ability to dial it up to 100 percent, but also are able to sit silently and calm their mind. Spiritually, they have the ability to tap into a higher power or motivation. In an age where people do not back up their words with action, Coach Divine lives the SEALFIT concepts he teaches. Not only is he extremely accomplished from a physical standpoint, he is both mentally and spiritually strong as well. Never content to sit and watch from the sidelines, Coach Divine leads from the front, showing by example that the needs of the team come before the needs of an individual and no person is too important to do the little things. This willingness to train and suffer with the group motivates everyone to raise their game.

Over the past 12 months, I have had the privilege of training under Coach Divine, and I have seen firsthand the effects that his SEALFIT program can have. Pre-Special Ops, military, LEO/First Responder trainees, and elite athletes become stronger and more mentally focused than they had previously thought possible. Weekend warriors break through barriers and prove to themselves the viability of Coach Divine's 20x principle that everyone is capable of 20 times more than they thought possible. The concepts presented in this book are not mere theory. They are concepts that have been proven and refined over the course of Coach Divine's 20-year career as a Navy SEAL, competitive athlete, martial artist, and business owner. If you have a desire to improve yourself, become a leader, and foster a warrior spirit in whatever arena you compete, *8 Weeks to SEALFIT* is going to give you the tools you need to succeed.

  —Joe L.
  SEALFIT athlete

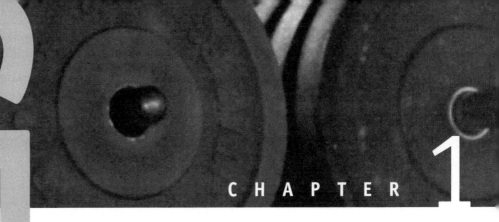

CHAPTER 1

EMBRACE
THE SUCK

YOU JUST SET FOOT ONTO THE NAVY SEAL'S BASIC UNDER-
WATER DEMOLITION/SEAL (BUD/S) TRAINING COMPOUND.
THE SUN'S BEATING DOWN. THE OCEAN BOOMS IN THE
DISTANCE. YOU ARE STANDING IN YOUR WORKOUT SHORTS, WHITE
T-SHIRT, AND COMBAT BOOTS, AND NERVOUS ENERGY TINGLES UNDER
YOUR SKIN. TAKING A FEW DEEP BREATHS, YOU PREPARE TO DEMON-
STRATE THAT YOU HAVE WHAT IT TAKES TO BE A SEAL.

The instructor eyes you like a piece of fresh meat and says, "Your first exercise is push-ups. Perform as many perfect, Navy SEAL–style push-ups as you can in two minutes. I will demonstrate."

He assumes the plank position, then lowers himself like a board until his chest touches the ground, then rises back up to full arm extension. The instructor then demonstrates the what-not-to-dos—no chicken dip, hip drops, or resting on your knees. You pair up with a swim buddy and hear, "Three, two, one, go!"

You complete your set, then rest 10 minutes. Next up is maximum repetitions of sit-ups in 2 minutes. Hands touching shoulders, elbows touch knees in the up position. Easy day, so far! Until you hit 50.

After sit-ups, another 10-minute break, then come the pull-ups. Do as many as you can before you gas out. You must get your chin over the bar in a strict dead-hang pull-up. No *kipping*—manipulating your hips to gain upward momentum.

Another 10-minute rest separates the pull-ups from the pool, where you complete a 500-meter swim using the combat sidestroke. Finally, a 1.5-mile run caps off the test. *Hooyah!* The first workout of BUD/S is in the bag. You realize, however, that this is just the beginning; there's a long road ahead. But you're up for the challenge, because you've trained in SEALFIT to prepare.

Welcome to 8 Weeks to SEALFIT!

You've chosen to show your instructor (me) that you have the stuff to be SEALFIT. Now suit up and get the baseline screening test done! That's right. You're doing what you just read. If you can't or won't do this, don't bother with the rest of the book. Put it down and walk away. I don't work with people who aren't ready to commit. When you're ready to continue, complete:

1.   as many perfect, Navy SEAL–style push-ups as you can in 2 minutes

2.   10-minute rest

3.   as many sit-ups as you can in 2 minutes

4.   10-minute rest

5.   as many pull-ups as you can before you gas out

6.   10-minute rest

7.   a 500-meter swim (or substitute a 2,000-meter row if you don't have access to a pool)

8.   10-minute rest

9.   a 1.5-mile run

10.   Record your repetitions and times in a journal!

Check online at www.sealfit.com/screeningtest to compare your results to the SEAL standards. Get it done. Then come back and read the end of this chapter. Good luck!

SEALFIT Training

SEALFIT TRAINING INVOLVES MORE THAN push-ups, sit-ups, pull-ups, running, and swimming. However, you'll use these key functional movements and a few others every day. If you hope to be SEALFIT, you have to be able to do the basics. No excuses. No quitting.

Navy SEALs do nothing unless it's critical. Everything they do in the gym or on the grinder (the large open space in the SEAL compound where the bodies, minds, and spirits of the candidates are ground down and then rebuilt) supports actual SEAL missions later on. You don't see SEALs working dumbbell curls, leg extensions, or any funky machines. All that they need is a body and a few simple tools: pull-up bar, rope, dip bar, set of free weights, kettlebell, sandbag, jump rope, and a few other odds and ends. They keep it simple. So do I. The screening test described on the previous page works because all the movements are functionally oriented toward key SEAL physical needs—pushing, pulling, running, swimming, and a strong core.

The baseline will smoke you if you put 100 percent into each evolution. It tests your capacity to do a lot of work in a short period of time—what I call *work capacity*. It reveals the efficiency of your muscles, or stamina. And it proves your endurance. Going full-out challenges your mental fortitude. You've tasted only a few of the domains that SEALFIT will develop to an entirely new level. As you progress, you'll be astounded at what I ask you to do, and what you find that you can do.

As in the actual Navy SEAL program, I aim to shock your system. I need to break you down so I can build you back up the SEALFIT way. In the meantime I need you to set aside any beliefs about what should and shouldn't be done, or what you can and can't do. I don't care whether you're a strongman or a skinny weakling; I've trained all types. If you commit to SEALFIT, we will transform you into a lifetime functional athlete. The secret is embracing the suck, every training session, day in and day out. As you habituate discipline and courage, SEALFIT will stop being hard. The suck will be fun. You won't want to live without it.

An "Average" 40-Year-Old Business Owner

Bobby spends most of his time riding a desk. After training in CrossFit for a year, he enrolled in my Unbeatable Mind Academy (UMA). UMA is an online mental toughness program that introduces SEALFIT training in a progressive manner, after some foundational mental skills are developed. Bobby jumped right into the SEALFIT Advanced Operator Training workouts after resolving to get serious.

Every workout crushed him. He would cuss at SEALFIT and me as he struggled with the 2-hour sessions—which made his former workouts seem like a warm-up. Most days he had to scale the loads and substitute for things he couldn't do. But Bobby embraced the suck. After 3 months a dramatic shift occurred.

The phone rang . . .

"Coach Divine," I said as I picked up the call.

"Coach . . . Bobby Yates here. . . . I called to tell you about a breakthrough!" He was clearly excited.

"For the last three weeks I have finally been able to complete the Advanced Operator Training workouts as prescribed. I didn't care if it took me three hours."

"Sounds like a great milestone, Bobby."

"But something amazing happened. My strength and performance suddenly improved dramatically. I've got this new sense of confidence I've never had. I went from dragging myself to workouts to now really looking forward to them." He was practically beaming into the phone.

"I got this swagger as I go about my day. I'm a machine at work and have tons of energy to spend with the family."

He finished with: "My friends think I'm crazy, but I feel stronger—physically and mentally—than I have in years. . . . I feel like I'm twenty again!"

Bobby had tapped into a secret of SEALFIT training. When we establish a new norm for the human experience, we step up to meet the challenge. Our bodies, minds, and spirits adapt. Bobby's new normal is very uncommon in the world today. That makes Bobby uncommon. He's no longer an average guy. He's someone special.

More Than a Workout Program

After 8 weeks of the SEALFIT training program, you will begin to:

- Work at near peak output for extended periods of time, with unknown rest periods.

- Prepare for the known and the unknown.

- Find a way to work out, whether or not you have access to a gym or the so-called proper training tools.

- Compete not only to win, but also to survive and accomplish a mission that has life, death, or strategic consequences well beyond your own pay grade.

- Be strong without being concerned about shows or competitions of strength.

- Possess stamina to move heavy objects around.

- Utilize exceptional endurance for completing long distances.

- Demonstrate an intense capacity for working in explosive, short bursts such as a firefight or other crises.

- Retain durability and powerful core strength, without as many injuries. You'll be knowledgeable about sustaining the body at high levels of readiness over a long haul.

- Profess mental toughness, understanding that training is required for that toughness.

See, SEALFIT is far more than a workout program. It's a way of life. It will change the way you see yourself. You'll become more confident and capable, demonstrating a mental fortitude that will allow you to dominate any challenge. You'll soon tell me what I heard the other day from Bobby Yates—"Coach Divine, I've changed."

It's your turn. Be someone special. Now get some rest. Tomorrow's gonna kick your ass.

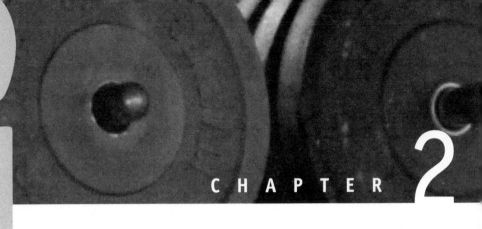

CHAPTER 2

FORGING A WARRIOR MIND-SET

NOW THAT YOU'VE COMPLETED THE BASELINE TEST, YOU PROBABLY THINK YOU'RE READY TO START TRAINING. NOT SO FAST. WE NEED TO PREPARE YOUR MIND TO BE AN ALLY, RATHER THAN AN ENEMY.

Welcome to Hell!

"Welcome to Hell!" says Instructor Zinke with a sideways smile. "Assume you're checking into Hotel Hell Week . . . or did you come to quit like the rest?"

Hell Week? Oh, yeah, you think to yourself. *I'm here for Hell Week, all right, and scared shitless.* "Yes, sir, I am here for Hell Week, and no, sir, you would have to kill me to get me to quit."

You instantly regret those words. Zinke stares right through you and says: "No problem, if that's what it's gonna take!"

Seventy teammates, out of 180 who started 7 weeks ago, remain. They shove gear in duffel bags, stencil T-shirts, and prepare themselves for the coming challenge.

Holy cow, I'm finally doing this. I'm about to jump into the abyss. Am I ready? you ask yourself.

After a few awkward jokes, your teammates retire to their racks for a final snooze before the games begin. Five days and nights of brutal, around-the-clock training. You sit on your rack to review your worn copy of *8 Weeks to SEALFIT*. Recalling that *kokoro* means "merging of heart and mind in action," you're going to need all the kokoro spirit you can muster. Coach Divine's words pierce your thoughts:

"Find a quiet place to prepare your mind."

An hour before it all begins you head to the beach . . .

The Mental Game

It's unusually quiet, the calm before the storm. You look beyond the waves and soften your eyes, slipping into the meditative state you learned at SEALFIT. After about 5 minutes of sitting and watching the waves roll in, you have reached a state in which your mind is still water running deep. You review the physical and mental milestones met in preparation for this moment. Hours upon hours of physical training from Basic, to Intermediate, to Advanced Operator Workouts. You're ready for this. You review what you know about Hell Week as if watching a movie in your mind. You see yourself strong, injury free, alert and ready to lead, ready to follow, never quitting. That's who you are! Next you review your strategy and tactics for winning:

- **WHAT'S MY ULTIMATE GOAL?** Not just to survive, but to thrive.
- **WHY DID I COME HERE?** To meet myself for the first time, and earn the honor of wearing the Trident.

- **HOW DO I EXPECT TO ACHIEVE THIS?** One ordinary moment at a time, using extraordinary effort.

- **WHAT RESOURCES DO I HAVE TO DRAW UPON?** My strong mind, my strong body, my indomitable spirit, and my teammates.

There's still time left. Good, I need it to "dirt dive" the event.

You picture yourself getting the crap beat out of you with your teammates on the grinder, smiling. Images of another Hell Week you saw on YouTube play in your mind for a reference point. Experiences at SEALFIT Kokoro Camp, where you instilled the warrior mind-set, flash before you. You're standing proud at the end of every evolution, helping your mates. You've gone 48 hours with no sleep, but your mind's still alert. Your body freezes in the ocean, but deep breathing controls your mental and physical responses. Gazing in the mirror 5 days later, you smile, bright-eyed. "Class, you are secured!" rings out as you embrace your surviving teammates in gratitude. A sense of euphoria and peace washes over you as you reach your visualized goals.

Time grows short. You "charge up" for what's to come, plugging into the electricity inside and all around you. *Tap into it,* you tell yourself. You'll channel it for use during the week by maintaining the proper mental state, as if tuning to a radio frequency. You start with box breathing and soon evoke images of peak moments from the past. Strong emotions of battles fought and victories won arise. A positive internal dialogue awakens. An energetic high washes over you. You drop anchor in these positive seas, reciting William Ernest Henley's line from his poem "Invictus"—"I am the master of my fate: I am the captain of my soul."

The Warrior Mind

You may be one of the few to experience what I described above, but chances are you aren't and won't, for good reason. It doesn't matter. Replace the words "Hell Week" in the text above with whatever challenge you face. Developing a warrior mind-set remains the same. You think differently from the common man or woman. On the outside they may look like you, but on the inside you're very different. The mental preparation for the warrior mind-set allows you to dominate any challenge you accept in life.

- Stay focused and relaxed, adaptable to the changing situation.
- Know that you are going to succeed—there will be no wondering.

- Tap into energy that lies deep inside you, allowing you to be capable of at least 20 times what you think you are.

- Control fear and turn stress into success.

- Keep goals very short, and be prepared for whatever comes your way.

- Find humor in the challenge through a positive attitude that keeps you and your team motivated.

- Be decisive and confident, a true leader.

YOUR MISSION . . .

The greater the obstacle, the more glory in overcoming it. —CONFUCIUS

Before each training session, you will perform what I call a pretraining standard operating procedure (SOP). This is the same procedure you will use for a big challenge; it would just take a little more time. Find someplace quiet where you won't be distracted. Review the workout description in detail. Understand the protocol and all the exercises before ever beginning. Is your training space set up properly? What's your strategy—are you going to go straight through or break up the workout? Going for a new best in the strength or work capacity segments? Have your towel, journal, pencil, and water bottle ready? What about fuel—what will you eat as you run dry? What's your specific goal for this session? Check in with all this and remind yourself why you're committed to SEALFIT training.

Now see yourself performing the workout as written, with any modifications you may need. See mission success in your mind's eye. Rehearse the whole thing with perfect form. Finally, activate deep breathing and charge your body with positive energy and emotions, as if you had just hit a new personal best or had a major breakthrough. Begin a positive internal dialogue, which you will maintain throughout the training session. Okay. Feel more ready now? Sally forth and dominate, warrior. Once you've completed the workout, read the rest of this chapter.

WARM-UP: Watch range of motion (ROM), drills, burpee, and air squat video (www.sealfit.com/videos) at SEALFIT's Web site and practice 25 squats.

WORK CAPACITY: 5 rounds for quality:

- 20x air squats

- 20x burpees

- 200m (meter) run

COOL DOWN: 1-mile jog and long stretch.

COACHING NOTES: You've done your baseline (Training Day 1). These next 5 training days will prepare you for the On-Ramp and Advanced Operator Workouts. They'll cover some basic ground and get your mind and body in the game. Don't skip them. Even if you've done them before, improving your technique will yield enormous results in your training. You don't have to do them sequentially—you can take a rest day or two, depending on your starting fitness level.

Perform the **air squat** with feet apart at shoulder width, heels firmly planted into the ground. Extend your arms directly in front of you and pretend someone is pulling on your wrists. Now push your bottom slightly backward and sit down without bending your back. Keep your lumbar arch engaged and tight, keep your heels firmly planted, get your hips below the knee line. Wiggle your toes to ensure your weight is on your heels. Stand up in an explosive movement and push your hips slightly into hyperextension. Full depth, open hips at the top, engaged lumbar arch, and firmly planted heels are the keys.

Start your **burpees** from the standing position. Drop your body vigorously to the ground by kicking your feet backward, land in the push-up position, and lower yourself with expedited speed until your chest is touching the ground. Explode from the ground to the standing position and conduct a 6-inch jump as well as clapping hands overhead 1 time.

This Is SOP

What you've just performed is the standard operating procedure (SOP) for mental preparation in SEALFIT training. SEAL teams use the same warrior mind-set techniques when preparing for dangerous real-world missions. True warriors through the ages have discovered this secret: You must win the first battle—in your mind—to win every other battle in life. Remember: SEALFIT is more than training the body. You must embrace the whole person and see yourself as a body-mind-spirit. You'll train these simultaneously, leading to optimal performance and greater success in all your endeavors.

We don't do "easy" at SEALFIT. Training the body is simple compared to training the mind. One of my favorite mantras is "Where the mind leads, the body follows." Lead your mind to victory that you can see, feel, and believe, and your body will follow you to hell and back.

SEALFIT mental preparation has four distinct steps, which will get trained at deeper levels as you progress through the program:

1. Clear your mind. Eliminate distractions and allow thoughts of daily thises and thats to fall away. Develop a deep, positive concentration on the task ahead of you.

2. Know your "why" and your strategy and tactics. Modify them if need be based on changing conditions.

3. See victory in your mind, and practice for it. SEALs use processes we call *envisioning* and the *dirt dive*.

4. Charge your internal batteries for optimal performance.

Note: See Appendix 1 for a detailed explanation of the pretraining and post-training SOPs, and daily rituals of SEALFIT.

The Four Basic Skills

Begin practicing these four basic skills immediately. Just as with physical workouts, the more you train, the more you'll improve:

1. **BOX BREATHING:** Begin to take control of your breathing. Later, this will allow you to control fear and stress and maintain a calm body and mind. SEALs call it *arousal control*. Simply start by exhaling all the air from your lungs, then breathing slowly into your belly to a count of 4. Hold your breath to a count of 4. Then exhale to a count of 4, expelling all the air at the end. Finally, hold your lungs empty for a count of 4. The 4–4–4–4 count is a *box*, hence the name of this drill. Do this breathing exercise before your training for at least 5 minutes.

2. **POSITIVE INTERNAL DIALOGUE:** What you say to yourself matters a lot. Though this skill can be quite difficult because internal dialogues can be pretty deeply

rooted, just start by paying attention to your thoughts, then overriding negative thoughts with positive ones. The statement I used during SEAL training was "Feeling good, looking good, oughta be in Hollywood!"

3. **VISUALIZATION:** What you see in your mind also matters a lot! You'll learn to rehearse in your mind, as well as visualize future outcomes you strongly desire. Start by visualizing your training session before you start. SEALs call this "dirt diving"!

4. **GOAL SETTING:** Having well-set goals fuels focus, direction, and momentum. When facing a monster challenge like Hell Week, reduce it to micro-goals. You can digest bite-size chunks of an elephant long before swallowing the whole thing at once.

I grew stronger during Hell Week those many years ago. My boat crew made it through as a team, winning every evolution and securing victory 3 hours early on Friday. Forging a warrior's mind had everything to do with it. Out of 180 who began, less than 40 finished. Mental training transformed my life. It's going to transform yours, too.

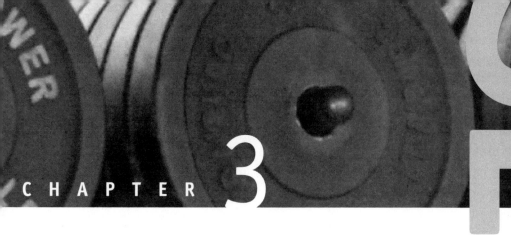

3

STAYING IN
THE FIGHT

NO REP!" SHOUTED COACH SMITH. "GET YOUR HIPS BELOW
PARALLEL ON THAT SQUAT. I THOUGHT YOU SAID YOU CAME
PREPARED. YOU'RE GONNA FAIL THIS BASELINE TEST
'CAUSE YOU DIDN'T TRAIN PROPERLY."

GOOD, I THOUGHT. *THAT'S HIS JOB. BREAK 'EM DOWN SO WE CAN BUILD
'EM UP.*

But we were only an hour into Kokoro Camp, and this guy was already struggling. Smith moved on to his next victim. But along came Coach Cummings.

"What do we have here, another quitter? Whatta ya here for? Why don't you just leave now? Open your hips at the top of the squat . . . no rep!"

The trainee stopped in his tracks, tore his shirt off, and launched it in Cummings's face. He stormed off and quit.

Watching from a short distance away I was stunned. No trainee attends Kokoro Camp without the preparation needed for success. I offer videos (www.sealfit.com/videos) that explain the purpose and intensity of the instructors, and how masterfully they exploit emotional weakness. Scratches and wounds get salted with barbs and verbal jabs, forcing trainees to persevere with inner resolve.

But we hadn't really started the hard part yet—this was just the baseline test. This trainee had lost total emotional control and quit the fight, leaving his teammates behind. Had he harnessed his emotions in that moment of choice, he would have survived the weekend and grown stronger from it. Now his lesson would linger with the pain of regret.

Let the Hammer Hit Your Funny Bone

Let's face it, life is tough. But it's tougher if you're stupid. When you don't prepare and don't learn from life's many challenges, that's stupid. By the way, have you ever stopped to consider how many disasters you've created in your life? How *you* respond makes the difference between heaven and hell. If you want to end the disaster cycle, learn to find grace and humor even in life's hardest challenges.

I say, "Let the hammer hit your funny bone." Rather than curl up and hunker down to ride out the storm, make light of the situation and find the lesson lurking inside. When I suffer during training, I shove a smile on my face and yelp the Howard Dean Scream (google it if you want a refresher or were too young to hear it). My team's sucking wind, too, and a sudden charge of humor shifts our group's emotional state. Soon we're laughing and hooting in our shared misery. You find great power when you remember that you're not alone.

When things got really bad in the SEAL teams, we'd say, "Time to put up or shut up." That meant: Make a positive contribution right now or shut your mouth. The most positive contribution was humor. To this day I have fond memories of the laughter during Hell Week. It truly became one of the funniest weeks of my life, because both the instructors and the students who survived understood humor's power to minimize the hardships of life. It develops grace through emotional control.

Lack of physical preparation had nothing to do with the Kokoro trainee who quit in the first hour. He quit because he lacked emotional control and resiliency. He couldn't find the humor or grace in his moment of choice. You're not a Kokoro quitter, are you?

Your Four Dominant Emotions

Today's first assignment: Grab your journal, sit quietly, and reflect upon which four dominant emotions drive your behavior. Do you operate out of fear? Anger? Jealousy? Love? Joy? Courage? Be brutally honest with yourself. No one's watching. Write your four down. It's very important. The Kokoro quitter operated out of anger and fear of failure. They defeated him.

Got your four down? Good. Now, answer the following questions:

1. What do these emotions keep me from creating in my life?

2. What beliefs create these four emotions?

3. What would I be like, and what would my life be like, if I could control these emotions?

Now we're getting somewhere. Next I want you to close your eyes, and envision four new ideal emotions that you strongly desire. Replace fear with courage, anger with joy, jealousy with acceptance, pessimism with trust. Whatever four emotions you originally chose to describe yourself, choose more positive emotions now. When you've written down your four, answer these questions:

1. What benefit would it bring me and others if I acted with these ideal emotions?

2. What beliefs do I need to change, and what new beliefs do I need to develop, to own these ideal emotions?

3. What would I be like and what would my life be like, if I replaced my original four dominant emotions with these four ideal emotions?

Reflect on your answers daily for the next 3 weeks. After 21 days your new beliefs and emotions will begin to form habits, which will define your new character.

Depth and Span

The depth and span of your emotional intelligence determines whether you stay in the fight and finish what you start or become a Kokoro quitter. We all churn with emotions, both positive and negative. How aware are you of their full complexity (depth) and range (span)? Do you have a healthy response to negative emotions, and a healthy expression of positive ones? Negative emotional responses derail you from your commitments. Poor emotional control limits your peak performance and forces you to suffer. Either your emotions manage you or you manage them.

Have you known anyone who possessed a brilliant mind, but whined like an emotional infant? I have. Some of my grad school professors fit that bill. How about a charismatic leader who let their emotions torpedo their career and reputation? Grab today's newspaper and pick an example!

Being SEALFIT requires an awareness of the depth and span of your emotional life. As your awareness deepens, you will manage emotional responses positively and develop powerful habits that forge emotional resiliency.

Develop Emotional Resiliency

Now that you've glimpsed mental toughness, here's what we're really after: emotional resiliency. Emotional resiliency is the power to bounce back when circumstances rain bricks on you. How have you responded when you lost your job, have been rejected by your first love, or made a crucial mistake on your taxes? Do you allow negative emotions to take hold and confuse your thinking? Or do you draw from a deep well of optimism?

Here are four steps to develop emotional resiliency. Your goal is not to just stay in the fight, but to crush it every time!

1. **SELF-CONTROL:** Start by developing the ability to witness and then control your emotional states. Emphasize positive emotions and eradicate uncontrolled responses to negative ones.

2. **SELF-ESTEEM:** Make habits of your four new ideal emotional states and develop your self-esteem in the process. Believe in your inherent goodness and value.

3. **OPTIMISM:** Start a daily focus on the positive things that happened and journal them nightly. Soon you will dig a deep well of optimism and drink from it daily.

4. **SELF AND OTHERS:** Learn to take care of yourself while *also* taking care of your teammates. This "self and others" focus will affect all areas of your life. You'll gain intrinsic worth and motivation from helping others and forget about being self-absorbed.

Your Mission . . .

WARM-UP: Watch butterfly sit-ups, kettlebell swings, and push-up videos (www.sealfit.com /videos). Then perform ROM drills, then 10 perfect reps of each exercise in work capacity.

WORK CAPACITY: Complete 21–15–9 reps as fast as possible, with great forms, of:

- butterfly sit-ups
- kettlebell swings
- push-ups
- 400m run after each set of repetitions

COOL DOWN: 1-mile walk or jog and long stretch.

COACHING NOTES: Hydrate and refuel. Journal your results. Perform 21 of each exercise, then 15 of each, then 9 of each.

Perform the **butterfly sit-up** with the soles of the feet placed together and close to the crotch. It better isolates the abdominal muscles and eliminates the stress on the hips and quads. Also don't brace your feet or place your hands behind your neck. Place them straight above your head with arms extended. Throw the arms forward and pull the body up into the sitting position. Sit all the way up and touch the toes with both hands. Placing a rolled-up towel or using an AbMat under the lumbar arch will greatly increase the success of this exercise.

Assume the **push-up** position with your knees off the ground. Lower yourself until your right cheek touches the ground and then rapidly explode upward until your arms are fully locked. Repeat touching the left cheek to the ground.

As you progress through today's workout, pay close attention to any emotions that arise and your natural response to them. Write them all down in your journal. Begin to control your emotional response as you also control your internal dialogue. Soon you'll change your overall state of being through a powerful combination of beliefs, body language, thoughts, and internal dialogue. You'll laugh at the thought of ever being a Kokoro quitter.

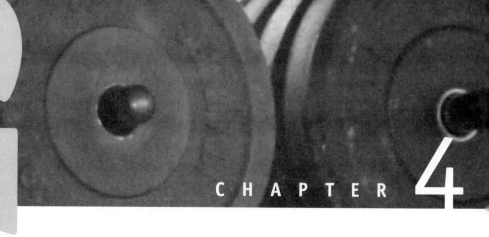

CHAPTER 4

TRAINING ISN'T "WORKING OUT"

MY SPINE TINGLED. A THOUSAND RHINOS POUNDED THE WALLS OF MY STOMACH. DARKNESS CLAWED ITS WAY ACROSS THE SKY. MY PLATOON AND I STRETCHED OUT LIKE A LINE OF ANTS ON THE SNOW-COVERED RIDGELINE. INSTEAD OF OPENING UP TO A PLATEAU, AS I THOUGHT THE MAP INDICATED, THE TERRAIN GREW STEEPER. A DEEP RAVINE WITH AN 800-FOOT DROP opened its teeth to the right of us. I watched Swanson struggle 20 yards above me. The plan had to change. . . . Too late!

"Shit, Cyborg, I lost my footing!" (Cyborg was my SEAL nickname.)

Swanson started to slide, then roll toward me. Every ounce of focus and years of physical training poised me like a tiger ready to pounce. I dug my ice ax into the rocky snow. He picked up speed and slammed into me like a truck. We tumbled toward the cliff, my team looking on helplessly.

As I grappled for control, a deep awareness I can describe only as *surreal flow* overrode my fear and slowed time to a standstill. I found my stomach and lay down on my ax, digging it into my chest as much as the hill. Mental focus controlled the pain as we jerked and bounced. We ground to a halt a mere foot from the abyss. My breathing was controlled and deep, my body calm as we lay there for a moment, relishing the new lease on life. Swanson looked over at me.

"Thanks, Cy, you saved my life . . . again!"

Time and again life as a SEAL plunged me into life-and-death situations. Awareness helped me to handle crisis after crisis with a calm, cool demeanor. They never allowed me time to think, and simply working out to prepare wouldn't have cut it. Yes, I was eminently fit and had a great plan, but had I not relied on a deep awareness to control my mind and breathing, the outcome would have been very different. These skills must be trained.

"SEALFIT LOOKS AWESOME, BUT I'M gonna work out at Gold's Gym a few more months to get in better shape first."

"Bill, training with us isn't working out. What you seek with SEALFIT you won't find at Gold's or anywhere else. I'm not trying to sell you, but in three months your plan will leave you exactly where you are today. Start SEALFIT now. In three months you'll be a different person."

"But SEALFIT looks really hard and I don't want to pay for two memberships."

"Okay, Bill, good luck, and give me a shout when you're ready to progress."

He slunk off. He had no focus, no plan, no idea what he really wanted beneath the push and pull of his usual reactions. I could lead a horse to water, but I couldn't make him drink. Ralph Waldo Emerson said that "when a man is pushed, tormented, defeated, he has a chance to learn something." Would Bill ever become aware of the chance that lay before him?

Two years later while eyeballing a banana at Seaside Market, I heard someone shout, "Hey, Mark!"

There stood Bill, older and rounder.

"Howzit going, Bill? Good to see you! How's your training?"

His body screamed the answer above any words he said. He was "working out," a surefire way to nowhere fast. Bill wasn't ready then. Will he ever be?

"Isn't This a Workout Book?"

No. It's serious training for serious people, like you.

"Then what's training?" you ask.

Training is passionately applying carefully conceived principles to develop yourself physically, mentally, and spiritually. It cultivates a deep awareness of your inner and outer worlds and aligns these worlds into a serious force. You show up as exceptional every day.

"*Sounds* different than working out," you say.

I hope so. Look more closely at the four key elements of a world-class training program.

PURPOSE-DRIVEN

No serious commitment happens without a rock-solid foundation and purpose. In my early 20s I literally thought my boring life was all there was. Then I found a mentor in Kaicho Tadashi Nakamura, master of Seido Karate. He taught me how to train my whole person. He honed the mental, emotional, and spiritual skills I needed to succeed as a SEAL. Joining the SEALs continued my journey to be a warrior and a better person every day. Now it's time for me to give back and mentor you on this path. My purpose with SEALFIT training is lifelong growth of your physical, mental, emotional, intuitional, and spiritual capacities.

Aligning yourself with this purpose will fuel your training over the short and long haul, as it has mine. Bill did not realize that no real purpose backed his efforts. He assumed that random appearances at a place like Gold's Gym would lead to fitness results. He wanders through the fitness wasteland, waiting for a treadmill to open up so he can dawdle time away watching TV while sweating a bit. If that's you, it's time to change.

Nothing good in life comes easily. The accomplishments you hold most dear require your most valiant efforts. The same holds true of SEALFIT. Your courage to start and your deep commitment to endure will strengthen you at all levels and shape you into a better person.

But first take a moment to answer the question: "Why am I training in SEALFIT?" It could be something external like "looking good on the beach," "losing weight," or "competing in the CrossFit Games." Or you might find a deeper purpose like "being the best husband and father possible" or "getting better every day and having optimal health." Which do you think will sustain you longer?

Write your answers in your journal. Get your purpose clear before reading any further. You'll need to tap into it when it's time to embrace the suck.

PASSION-FILLED

Passion is more than sex and ice cream. It can even be something painful like training. Passion lights your hair on fire with enthusiasm toward a worthy pursuit. It doesn't let you continue your pretend game of working out, like Bill. You need all you can to apply to your training. Here's how:

- **FIND THE FUN.** For me, fun is team camaraderie, the exhilaration of performing difficult tasks well, and the joy of learning something new. What is it for you? Recognize and love the simple, good things in life so much they make you laugh, cry, or both together. Now plug the same level of passion into your training.

- **APPRECIATE THE HARD.** You may never love pain, soreness, occasional injuries, or the feeling of defeat, but you can certainly learn to value the lessons these inevitable roadblocks bring. Consider them part of training and life. Deal with them well, learn to appreciate them, and you'll soon discover a growing emotional resiliency.

- **FOCUS DAILY.** Develop a disciplined habit of training. Even your rest days count. Be steady, week in and week out. Training, eating, and breathing are the three pillars of optimal health, so master them now! Don't bump a training session without serious thought. If you must, make it up. When you travel, you train. When it snows, you train. When you're injured, you train. Got it?

- **MEASURE YOUR PROGRESS.** Many of you have worked with a private trainer who tracked your progress. Good, but it's better for you to track your own progress and then celebrate it. In SEALFIT you'll track and benchmark your progress daily and weekly, noting your steady, forward march.

- **GROW.** Don't buy into the broken belief that younger is better. Don't be a Bill and decay with time. I feel stronger and better now at 50 than I did at 30. Take control. Learn to grow. You're adding new skills, knowledge, and awareness in an upward spiral toward virtuosity. Soon you'll think like a kid again. The world is your playground!

PRINCIPLE-BASED

SEALFIT training anchors its roots in solid principles that will pass the test of time. I've tested and proven them to work for anyone. Thousands upon thousands have improved their lives through SEALFIT—1,200 have survived the rigors of Kokoro Camp to date. I've kept the principles that worked and discarded all else from my own experience with endurance sports, powerlifting and Olympic lifting, Navy SEAL training, P90X, TRX, yoga, Pilates, CrossFit, multiple forms of martial arts, and even a few aerobics classes. Here are a few:

- **STRENGTH DEVELOPMENT** (not bodybuilding) builds a foundation of durability. SEALFIT implements the strength-building techniques of powerlifting, Olympic lifting, and strongman models. They build confidence in you and your team, particularly in a crisis. If you don't need a team, don't expect a crisis, and are a superhero with no weaknesses, avoid them.

- **FUNCTIONAL MOVEMENT** allows your body to move as is intended by your creator. SEALFIT draws from CrossFit, yoga, martial arts, and Navy SEAL training, and augments these with some innovations of our own.

- **STAMINA AND WORK CAPACITY** keep you in the fight when things get tough.

- **ENDURANCE TRAINING** ensures you can go the long haul.

- **DURABILITY AND MENTAL TOUGHNESS** allow you to avoid injury, train though injury, and stay the course over a lifetime.

These defining principles, along with others, will unfold in greater detail in the pages to come. You won't identify with Bill ever again.

PLANNED CAREFULLY

When you played sports in high school, you didn't just flail around on the field. A coach guided you according to a plan. At a yoga or martial arts studio you don't just do what you want. Your teacher instructs you with strategic insight. It's the same in exercise and nutrition. Being your own health and fitness coach is a flailing waste of time.

In this book, I am your head coach. You may find another coach to work with you in person. Just make sure that you find one who understands and agrees with the principles in this book. If not, you're in for a confusing time.

8 weeks to SEALFIT training is:

- **PROGRAMMED** to balance strength, stamina, work capacity, endurance, and durability.
- **PERIODIZED** training to cycle through phases of shifting emphasis to allow recovery.
- **POWERED WITH FUEL** so that you view food as an integral part of your training. You can't feed a Maserati with Yugo fuel.
- **PRIORITIZED** to focus your efforts into what's important in your life. It will slingshot you in a new direction and plug you into the SEALFIT lifestyle.

One final point: SEALFIT is **flexible!** I don't expect nor do I want perfection. I call it the 80–20 rule. Seek to perform 80 percent of your planned training and fueling goals. Allow a 20 percent buffer for spontaneous days off from training and cheat days with meals. Life is too short to be rigid and boring. Enough theory. Let's train.

Be Aware and Breathe

As you may now know, I take breathing very seriously. I know it sounds silly. Everyone breathes. But it amazes me how many people never think about their breathing. Something so important to life requires at least a momentary thought. I'm going to help you learn as much as you can about it . . . and even master it.

Really?? Can we get to the f#@%ing workouts already!

Slow down. Take a breath, my friend. Gaining deep awareness and control of your breath is one of the most essential tools in life. It's a secret practice of ancient yogis and martial artists to develop more power, presence, and mental control.

I introduced you to box breathing in chapter 2. Now I'm giving you more breathing principles and tips for your training sessions. Put them to work immediately in today's workout. Here are your marching orders:

BREATHING: THE SEALFIT WAY

1. Before your training session, perform the box breathing exercise for 5 minutes. This will ground you, clear any baggage from your mind, and energize you for the work ahead.

2. As you begin your session, put your attention back on your breathing pattern. Lengthen and deepen your breathing. Your mind will remain focused and you will relax into the pain as it enters your conscious awareness, which won't take long!

3. During the entire session keep your breathing deep and diaphragmatic, even when winded. Try to press air deep into your lungs at the end of each inhale by pressing your belly out. In through your nose and out through your nose. You can exhale through the mouth if you need to speed up the rate of respiration.

4. When conducting low-intensity work (when your heart rate is not above 50 percent max effort) add a short hold at the top of your breathing pattern. Times to do this include long- and slow-distance endurance, or short but low-intensity stamina work.

5. During high-intensity training, such as sprints or a timed interval workout, try not to inhale through your mouth. If you feel you aren't getting enough air, use your mouth to take a few extra gulps of air and then go back to nostril breathing. Unlike breathing through your mouth, breathing through your nose stimulates the arousal control response. It cleanses and warms the air and also allows deeper, more penetrating breaths into your diaphragm.

6. When you reach an interval or a stop point in a session, come back to your deep,

rhythmic breathing and seek to completely relax your mind and body. Maintain total present moment awareness on your breathing. Breathe into the next set.

7. Regulate rest periods during interval training with a predetermined number of deep breaths. For instance, if you're doing 100 kettlebell swings, and your goal is to break at 20 reps, when you set the kettlebell down, commit to 5 deep breaths. As you breathe, bring total relaxation awareness into your body. Turn your attention inward, not worrying about anyone else, and just visualize slowing your heart rate and regulating your systems. Five breath cycles isn't a long time, but it activates your recovery mechanisms and deepens your presence. In presence you'll find more power and peace of mind in the midst of the pain and pressure. Over time you'll learn how to recover rapidly by maintaining a meditative focus on your breath, completely relaxing your body and literally willing it to recover.

YOUR MISSION . . .

WARM-UP: Watch rowing and box jumps videos (www.sealfit.com/videos). Then perform ROM drills, then 50 air squats, then 25 tuck jumps (knee to chest).

WORK CAPACITY: 5 rounds for quality and time of:

- 15x box jumps (20 or 24 inches)
- 18x sit-ups
- 20x air squats
- 500m row (substitute 500m sprint if you do not have a rower)

COOL DOWN: jog or walk 1 mile. Stretch or SEALFIT Yoga (see chapter 7).

COACHING NOTES: Hydrate, refuel, and journal results. This workout is about sustained workload across a broad time domain. It should take you around 30 minutes. Do your best to maintain the same pacing throughout all rounds. You don't want to use all your energy in the beginning, but you also don't want to save it until the end. The box jump is great for building strong bones and explosive power. Scale the height so you're certain you won't miss and ding your shin (a common occurrence at SEALFIT headquarters). When you land on top of the box, open your hips and stand completely erect. There is a plyometric version of the box jump, but I want you to learn to open your hips all the way because it's essential for the Olympic lifts you'll learn later on. It doesn't matter whether you jump or step down.

WELL DONE. JOURNAL YOUR EXPERIENCE. Note the difference that breathing and awareness made. You've begun to train for a purpose. When crises unleash their screams, you'll look them in the eye without flinching. You'll summon courage from deep within and watch as your body does what you command. You'll never go back to just "working out" again. If only Bill was ready to join us.

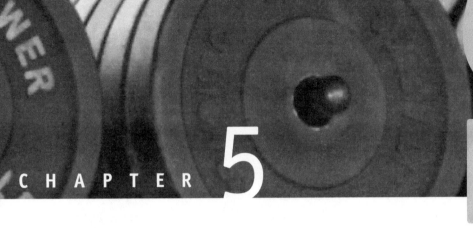

CHAPTER 5

THE FIVE MOUNTAINS

I WANT TO COME OUT FOR A WEEK TO TRAIN."

KYLE BASS WAS PERSISTENT. ORIGINALLY SEEKING A SEAL TO ASSIST WITH PERSONAL SECURITY, KYLE WANTED TO EXPER-IENCE THE REAL DEAL HIMSELF. *WELL NOW, WOULDN'T THAT BE A KICK IN THE PANTS,* I THOUGHT. REFLECTING ON MY OWN EXPERIENCE, I REALIZED MY MOST VALUABLE TRAINING CAME FROM IMMERSION EVENTS WHERE I ATE, BREATHED, SLEPT, AND TRAINED WITH A TEAM for an extended period, BUD/S being the most extreme example. It was there that my heart and mind merged with my actions.

This kokoro spirit didn't just help me survive BUD/S. It enabled me to lead other SEALs. Through twenty years as a Navy SEAL I felt it had guided me in every mission. Now Kyle wanted what I'd received from my mentors so many years ago.

Do I have what it takes?

Time slowed. I allowed thoughts and feelings inside me to voice their opinions.

Reintroducing a warrior-monk style of training to the West appeals to me. You learn fast when you engage your whole person. You develop at the physical, mental, emotional, and spiritual levels. I really want to do this for Kyle as a test, and then roll it out for elite military and professional athletes. My spark's lit, I'm game!

"Okay, Kyle, you're on," I said. "Be here Sunday at three p.m. prepared for anything and everything!"

SEALFIT Academy was born.

The Academy

My SEAL experience provided a reference point for what the human body could take. During Navy SEAL Hell Week (6 days of training with 4 total hours of sleep) I recall an instructor telling me, "You're capable of twenty times more than you think you are." Those words meant more to me after Hell Week as I reflected in awe at what the survivors had accomplished. The class began with 180 trainees and ended with 40 after Hell Week. The workload we endured simply wasn't humanly possible. But, amazingly, it was.

I wasn't sure how much I could throw at a civilian like Kyle. So I started timidly—only 10 hours a day for Kyle and his team, interrupted by meals. I even let them sleep! In the future, I pushed the envelope much further, searching for new methods to help them achieve that elusive 20x factor. I'm still searching.

Four years after the trial run with Kyle, a day in the life of SEALFIT Academy looked like this:

- 0500–0630 meditation and yoga
- 0700–0900 Advanced Operator Workout
- 0930–1100 LSD (long slow distance) team run
- 1100–1200 body control clinic

- 1300–1430 strength and power clinic

- 1500–1600 team development training

- 1600–1800 mental toughness lecture and drills

- 1800–1900 functional high intensity training

- 2100–2200 reading, contemplation, and journaling

- 2200 lights out

- 2400–0300 warrior spirit training

- 0500 wake, rinse, repeat

With no stone left unturned, the modern equivalent of the Spartan Agoge or civilian SEAL training took flight. Our 90 percent success rate with SEAL candidates satisfied my goal to inoculate trainees against failure in special-ops training. But the real reward has been with "average" folks who leave with a new lease on life and an unconquerable spirit.

SEALFIT Academy is human alchemy. The trainees arrive with a deer-in-the-headlights look, terrified of the unknown that lies ahead. Some disappear, never to show their faces on the grinder Monday morning. Those that endure Day 1 emerge euphoric and astonished. Then Day 2 comes, and then 3. Training is relentless. Something changes around Day 4—body, mind, and spirit adapt to the new reality. Fear is obliterated, replaced with excitement as personal power explodes. Trainees attack each evolution with positive enthusiasm. Breakthroughs occur one after another. The class unites as an elite team, opening up the 20x vista that goes beyond individual performance. I watch them climb the five mountains of human potential—physical, mental, emotional, awareness, and spirit—one footstep at a time.

Excited by the level of transformation I witnessed, I began to study human performance in other domains. I created a performance accelerator through an immersive journey into the ancient secrets of the master warriors. It challenged the modern warrior on multiple levels simultaneously, synthesizing and fueling growth faster than ever before. Worldviews and belief systems transformed alongside the Five Mountains.

The Five Mountains

The five primary human potentials, or "Mountains," that must be developed for warriors and leaders to operate at their peak are:

- Physical control and development
- Mental toughness and development
- Emotional awareness and resiliency
- Awareness and intuition
- Kokoro spirit

I advised you in the first chapter that SEALFIT is more than a fitness program. It's *integrated life training,* addressing all five of these Mountains as you progress. The net result: You develop in a balanced, accelerated manner—fostering significant breakthroughs in all areas of your life simply as the result of your training.

The Ten Domains of Mastery

Though this book primarily focuses on the first Mountain of physical development, you'll develop the other four, if you so desire. The information and drills in chapters 2 through 4 will guide your training for the subtler peaks of mental, emotional, and awareness development. The fifth Mountain, kokoro spirit, arises through crucible challenges such as the SEALFIT Kokoro Camp.

As you travel the Five Mountain path, ten skills define the way you act in performance. I call these the Ten Domains of Mastery. You can use them to grow no matter who you are or where you start on the journey. Let's explore them briefly. (Please join me in the Unbeatable Mind program to work on these in depth!)

1. **ENDURANCE:** One of four *foundational skills.* The other skills depend on it. You must develop this and the other three first.

   - At the physical level, you develop endurance when your body makes a habit of going long, in distance or time, powered by your extremities. A long run, ruck hike, swim, row, or bike ride constitutes an endurance event. These events rely on oxygen as fuel. People often refer to them as *cardio* because endurance trains the cardiorespiratory system to be more efficient.

   - At the mental and emotional level, endurance means that you develop the capacity to stay at a task for the long haul. Getting a black belt, finishing college, and becoming a SEAL all take mental and emotional endurance.

It requires mental, emotional, and spiritual endurance to raise a child or provide hospice care for a parent. You must master this critical skill to live life well.

2. **STRENGTH:** The second foundational habit. This is your ability to overcome resistance.

   ■ At the physical level you'll reap many benefits from good strength training. In the words of my strength mentor Mark Rippetoe: "Strong people are harder to kill than weak people, and more useful in general." I agree. But failure at most things is rarely the result of physical weakness alone. The stronger you are mentally, emotionally, and spiritually, the more successful and inspired you will be to maintain that overall strength. Why? So you can be more useful and have more fun in life, of course!

3. **STAMINA:** The third of the foundational habits. This allows you to overcome resistance, time and again. Pick something up or get hit—again, and then again. If you can do this gracefully for an extended period of time, you have stamina.

   ■ Mental stamina is associated with resiliency and your ability to maintain focus in the midst of chaos and fatigue. Emotional stamina is the resiliency that comes from bouncing back quickly from setbacks. Clearly you want this skill.

4. **FLEXIBILITY:** The fourth and final foundational habit, and the one often overlooked in training. In physical movements it leads to fuller ranges of motion, efficiency, and the avoidance of injuries.

   ■ "Semper Gumby" is the term we used in the SEALs to express developing a flexible attitude so we could ebb and flow with the changes that occur in fast-paced environments. Look around you. Fast-paced environments are the new normal.

5. **POWER:** The ability to overcome resistance *explosively,* such as snatching 185 pounds.

   ■ You can view physical power as *strength speed.* How fast can you accelerate a load from a dead stop to overhead? You can develop it with ballistic movements such as kettlebell swings or Olympic lifts.

- You develop mental power through concentrated focus on a task while accelerating your learning of the skills associated with that task.

- Emotional power develops when you connect with your heart and leverage the power of a team. Expressed in a crisis, it's often viewed as leadership.

6. **SPEED:** The rapid repetition of low-resistance loads. Most people don't need to be Speedy Gonzales, but developing speed leads to more confidence. It's useful in certain situations.

- You can increase your running speed by accelerating the cycle rate of picking up your feet and putting them down. Pose running is effective at developing speed with less energy output (www.sealfit.com/videos).

- Mental speed means you can take appropriate actions quickly because you've learned to discern truth and apply it rapidly to your decisions. Decisiveness requires clarity of thought and dexterity in communications. The Observe, Orient, Decide, Act (OODA) loop is the decision tool I teach for this skill.

7, 8, 9, and 10. **ACCURACY, AGILITY, COORDINATION, AND BALANCE:** You develop the final four domains as the result of neurological adaptation to practicing skills. Another way is to go outside and play in the real world—*functional training*. On mental, emotional, and spiritual levels, these last four domains are crucial for elite performance.

Respect

When I was young, I literally ran up the Adirondack Mountains in Upstate New York for the exercise and exhilaration. No doubt it fueled my ego to race past other plodding hikers. "Look at me! Aren't I amazing?" my actions screamed. As I revisit the mountains over the years I gain more and more respect for them. Respect literally means to revisit or take another look at something. As you train in your Five Mountains, day in and day out, you will revisit them again and again. As you see them from different perspectives, you will gain great respect for them and for yourself. When you respect yourself, you will respect others more deeply. The spiral of growth and success personally and socially spins upward.

Learn to appreciate the journey as much as the destination. I'm amazed by what I missed in the Adirondacks those early days. Walking the same trails, breathing the air, enjoying the trees and rich wildlife is like reading an entirely new book. The more you respect your training, the more competence and momentum you'll build.

"Slow Is Smooth, Smooth Is Fast"

In the SEALs, every new skill is introduced with a lecture, then slow, hands-on practice under the instructor's watchful eye. This is the "crawl" phase of the training, where we reinforce accuracy. Later we revisit the skill and practice a bit faster. We manage risk and assess feedback in this "walk" phase. Finally, after hours of "crawling and walking," we relished the freedom of exploding in the "run" phase. Competence had evolved from *unconscious incompetence* (pretraining), to *conscious incompetence* (crawl stage), then to *conscious competence* (walk phase), and finally to *unconscious competence* (the run phase, a precursor to mastery).

The experience is comparable to learning how to shoot a firearm. The first few times at the firing range, you fire with poor method and control. Shot patterns are all over the place. You have to slow down to control your body and mind in the simple act of pulling the trigger. Soon, though, your competence improves. You can now shoot out the bull's-eye. But you get cocky thinking you're Chuck Norris. So your shot pattern goes to hell and most of your rounds miss the target entirely.

Physical training is no different. You avoid the painful lessons by activating this mantra: *Slow is smooth, smooth is fast.*

Momentum

Select a training pace that's between slow and fast. Be methodical, purposeful, and maintain a relaxed awareness. Resist the urge to rush things. Breathe slowly and deeply. Your skill and accuracy will improve greatly. This is your efficiency zone where you can move at acceptable speeds and still be accurate, efficient, and effective. You can inch up the intensity as you improve this efficiency zone. It's an art born of personal experience. Patient training at this level of awareness leads to serious momentum.

If you go out at 100 miles per hour and get frustrated, you'll lose faith and fall off. You might have a few weeks of little or no training. When the frustration with your laziness hits a peak, you go out and crush yourself with intensity. Your next-day pain makes you give it up for another 3 weeks. In this scenario, you lack momentum. Bouncing between "zero" and "hero" leaves you no better off than when you were just working out.

Slow is smooth, smooth is fast. One day, 1 rep at a time. Soon you'll have 8 weeks of solid training days behind you. You'll scarcely notice an off or bad day. Serious momentum will fill you with discipline, drive, and determination. It will affect all of your Five Mountains and bring you success in other areas of your life. The upward spiral spins faster.

Okay, let's get to today's training session. **Maintain a focus** not just on the physical, but also on your mental, emotional, awareness, and spiritual aspects. Journal what you discover. Good luck!

THE FIVE MOUNTAIN MISSION

Pain is weakness leaving the body. —NAVY SEALS

WARM-UP: Watch grinder PT (physical training) intro and do warm-up (www.sealfit.com /videos). Then do pretraining SOP and ROM drills.

WORK CAPACITY AND STAMINA: Grinder PT—1, 2, or 3 rounds of the following as fast as possible with good form:

- 10x run and drop
- 10x DB (dumbbell) squat jumps (20–40-pound dumbbells)
- 20x push-ups
- 20x leg levers
- 15x burpees
- 15x 4-count smurf jumping jacks
- 15x tuck jumps
- 20x DB thrusters (front squat followed by a push press in 1 flowing motion)
- 20x push-ups (narrow)
- 20x crisscross jumping jacks

COOL DOWN: 1-mile jog or walk. Stretch or SEALFIT yoga.

COACHING NOTES: Journal your results. This is your first grinder PT session—try 2 or 3 rounds as a goal. If you simply can't handle the load yet, stop at 1 or 2. The grinder is an open training space at the Navy SEAL BUD/S training command, mirrored at our SEALFIT headquarters (HQ) compound. On it we "grind down" and rebuild character. It looks like a relatively simple body weight training session on the surface. When led by trained instructors, it quickly becomes a team crucible with a heavy mental toughness component. Here you'll use grinder PT to develop work capacity, stamina, and core strength. Grinder PT sessions occur for 20 to 45 minutes every Wednesday of advanced training.

At HQ, grinder PT can include any exercise or drill that the coaches conceive on the fly. A classic example of our grinder sessions includes the "deck of cards" workout where each suit is an exercise, the face value being the rep count. Flip a card, do the number of the exercise prescribed (aces high, jack, queen, and king are 11, 12, 13, and 15 respectively). The best grinder PT sessions are improvised by an inspired coach and fed by the team's energy. Typical exercises include jumping jacks, push-ups of all variations, sit-ups of all variations, pull-ups, leg levers, flutter kicks, wave-offs, mountain climbers, 8-count body builders, burpees, squats, lunges, jumping lunges, bear crawls, prisoner walks, and more.

CHAPTER 6

SEAL FUEL

EARLY IN MY SEAL TEAM DAYS I SURVIVED ON PIZZA, MILK, AND AN OCCASIONAL BEER. (WELL, OKAY, YOU GOT ME ON THAT ONE. THE BEER FLOWED LIKE A RIVER.) IT WAS THE CLASSIC BACHELOR DIET—GOOD ONLY FOR ITS CONVENIENCE. MY PERFORMANCE SUFFERED IMMENSELY. I FELT LIKE CRAP WHEN I WOKE UP. AFTER A 2-HOUR WORKOUT I FELT BETTER BUT THEN CRASHED AFTER LUNCH. MY ENERGY RODE A ROLLER COASTER. IF NOT FOR THE immense number of calories I burned daily, I would have exhibited the outward signs. I don't know how my insides survived.

It took a 6-month deployment to the Philippines and Guam to get my system back on track. I ate like the locals: fish and chicken—all range fed or hand caught, lots of vegetables, and some rice. I drank copious amounts of water to keep hydrated in the stifling heat. I noted how healthy I felt, and how healthy the citizenry appeared. This early experience with SEAL fueling changed my beliefs and habits forever.

Fast-forward to January 2009.

"Hi, Michael. Interested in the SEALFIT lifestyle?" My staff had fielded the caller's first twenty questions. They gave up and handed the phone to me. Michael was a Washington, D.C., lobbyist dabbling in martial arts. He wanted to scratch his "warrior itch" by attending a 3-week SEALFIT Academy and Kokoro Camp the following year.

"Tell me about yourself: training background, habits. What's your fueling plan?" I wanted to know his key indicators—food, fitness, and attitude. I can help him change the first two. The third he needed to bring to the table.

"I'm not functionally fit and eat like crap . . . I know I can do better . . . I really want to learn, but I'm clear across the country and so busy," he answered.

Within days Michael began training with a SEALFIT coach and following the program in this book. I wanted him to get his feet wet before I had the "come to Jesus" talk about nutrition. I knew he'd bounced around multiple "feeding plans" and used supplements. I tested the waters. He was willing to listen. *Sorta.* Back in 2009 our fuel plan required a leap of faith!

"No grains or milk!?" he asked.

Silence.

And then: "How can I train at such a high tempo and not eat grains or dairy?"

"Michael, set aside every conventional idea about nutrition you learned in school or picked up like an old boot along the way. SEALs are unconventional; we always look for what works and shit-can what doesn't. The conventional high-carb, low-fat diet is bull and causes most of the health problems we face in our society."

He kept listening.

"Carbs and sugar spike insulin, the fat-storing hormone. Grain processes just like sugar. And sugar-laden processed food leads to insulin disorders ranging from hypoglycemia to all-out diabetes. It opens the door to a host of other problems, including excess fat! Go caveman. Remove the sugar and grains. Your metabolism will rebalance. And fat, instead of being stored as excess adipose, will become the powerful source of fuel it was meant to be."

"But I avoid the foods with additives, preservatives, and coloring agents. Why do I have to give up grains and milk? What about bread, cereal, and pasta? Doesn't milk give you vitamin D and calcium? What about carb loading for big events? What about cholesterol risk?" he countered.

I let the protests run in one ear and out the other. I couldn't change years of mental programming in one conversation. "Michael, *I'm* a caveman. If you want to succeed at a high level, you'll have to think like a caveman, too. Thirty days on our fueling plan'll put hair on your chest and a furrow in your brow. You'll transform your health and vitality."

He grudgingly agreed. I let that beast lie for the next 2 months. I was just about to e-mail him when my cell phone rang.

"Coach Caveman!" It was Michael. "The changes in my body . . . my performance. I haven't touched grain or milk products in forty-five days. I feel great!"

"*Hooyah,* bro."

"I've already lost fifteen pounds and replaced it with muscle. My mind seems clearer, too. My energy's stable throughout the day. I just feel healthier. My lungs aren't congested. My stomach isn't bloated."

"Wow. Impressive list of side effects for a newly minted caveman."

We talked a few minutes longer before hanging up. I've seen people's bodies respond like Michael's so many times. That's what happens when you go "all-in" on SEAL fueling. Things change, for the better. Here's how . . .

Three Rules for Proper Fueling

Though I tried shocking Michael with my caveman statement, the truth is often stranger than fiction. SEAL fuel really is a caveman diet. It is commonly called the Paleo Diet. (Sometimes I even talk like a caveman.) In 2009 this diet had just gained some traction in the warrior communities through the work of Dr. Loren Cordain and his student, my friend Robb Wolf. (See www.RobbWolf.com.)

SEAL fuel's modified Paleo Diet comes from the presumed meal plan of the Paleolithic era. Without food storage, humans would have consumed the wild plants and animals that grew seasonally, when the "store" was open. No factories existed to cook, preserve, and freeze it. You had to eat it before it decayed naturally. In Caveman-speak: "Fresh food make good caveman."

Today you can generally find caveman food on the outer aisles of the grocery store. What foods are "game," so to speak? Protein sources include lean meats like fish, poultry, and wild game. Complex carbohydrates and more protein come from leafy green vegetables, nuts, seeds, and fruit. Perhaps the most valuable food source is good fat—from meats, nuts, and oils.

Paleo rules out packaged, processed foods; dairy; and any kind of grains, starches, and legumes (mostly beans, peas, lentils, and the like, but also extending to peanuts, which aren't technically nuts). "You not eat! Cooking, you can. Curing and preserving method with salt and chemical, not make happy." :-(

Okay, back to modern-day English. Based on my experience with SEALFIT athletes, here are my three Paleo modifications:

Mod 1: "80–20"—Warriors and SEALFIT athletes are adventurers and often find themselves in remote and random places. It's tough to eat the perfect meal while staying in a tent on Denali or even at home with the folks over the holidays. Sometimes an MRE is it, and boy, will it taste good. I propose an 80–20 rule. Stick to SEAL fuel Paleo style 80 percent of the time. Don't sweat the rest. Your metabolism will be firmly rooted in fat-burning mode. The occasional grain and sugary food won't upset the balance.

Mod 2: "More carbohydrates"—You'll be working harder than the average person with this program. A strict high protein, low glycemic diet, such as the Paleo, may lead to glycemic burnout. To avoid that, cycle more carbohydrates into your plan than those purely from vegetable sources. This works well with the 80–20 rule if your 20 percent is a cheat day every fifth day or so.

Mod 3: "Rice and beans"—My buddy Robb would say no. I say, "Go for it and note how you feel." Beans are a legume. Rice is a grain. But entire races thrive on these to add carbohydrates and bulk to their meat and veggies. These folks live long and prosper. I don't like being an absolutist in anything, especially when it comes to eating.

You can't stick to a fueling plan if it's too rigid. Personally, I also sneak milk every once in a while. I'm not lactose intolerant, and milk can be a ready source of protein in a shake after a hard training session. The point here is to be sensible. In Caveman: "Too much rigidity leave poor taste in mouth. Get clubbed by Paleo Diet."

"Okay, Mark, I believe you now, but what's the bottom line—how do I become a caveman fast?" you ask.

Good question. Let's get specific.

Five Steps to SEAL Fueling

Hint: Keeping a food journal side by side with your training journal helps, especially when starting out. Check out my SEALFIT training journal, which has much of this information, as well as journal pages for you at www.shop.navyseals.com.

STEP 1: Eliminate sugar and junk food, including any highly processed crud laden with additives and preservatives (sugar, soda, high-fructose corn syrup, MSG, aspartame, etc.). This will be difficult if you don't do steps 1 and 2 together.

STEP 2: Remove grain-based products from your diet 80 percent of the time. As mentioned, these include cereals, breads, and pastas. You'll have some withdrawal symptoms from steps 1 and 2—stand by! Replace these foods with more fresh vegetables, seasonal fruits, nuts, and seeds. Make sure that you enjoy the taste of most of these. Otherwise you'll pine for the days when you used to eat food that tastes good.

STEP 3: Eliminate cow's milk and highly processed cheeses and yogurts. If your health is fine and you don't have any negative responses to dairy, it's okay to reintroduce whole milk (20 percent of the time), raw cheese, and minimally processed, high-fat yogurt later on. You'll learn to like coconut and almond milk, among the other wonderful Paleoish products popping up these days.

STEP 4: Eliminate most starches and legumes (white potatoes, corn, beans, etc.). Use vegetables and seasonal fruits as your primary sources of carbohydrates, including sweet potatoes. Rice is also okay on a 20 percent limited basis.

STEP 5: Remove processed vegetable oils. Instead use olive oil for low-heat cooking and coconut oil for higher heat cooking. Avocados are an excellent source of good fat, as are walnuts and almonds.

I've included a shopping list in **Appendix 3** to help you choose the best SEALFIT fuel possible.

One final note about when to feed: The caveman ate when food was available. Three square meals a day is a myth. Vary your eating times and eat smaller meals throughout the day. Additionally, strive to refuel within 20 minutes of a strength or high-intensity training session. Missing this opportunity will lead to you turning from caveman to cannibal. Your muscles will literally cannibalize themselves in their manic hunt to replace depleted amino acids.

Now, unless you have further questions, it's time to put some hair on your chest (sorry, ladies). Here's an assignment to accompany today's training session. Good luck with your fueling plan.

Fuel Assignment

What's your attitude toward fueling? Grab your journal and write your responses:

- Do you break bread with others to build the team, or do you scarf fast food in a rush to get to your next appointment?
- Are you aware of where your food comes from or does it not matter?
- Is food simply nourishment for your body, or does it also nourish your mind and spirit?
- Do you wolf down your food wondering if your caveman neighbor is going to steal it, or do you actually taste and enjoy it?

Now, unless you're certain of what food you eat, tracking your intake will provide powerful insights. Often you understate the amount and overstate the quality of the foodstuff you cram into your system.

TRACK YOUR DAILY INTAKE FOR 1 WEEK

- When and where did you eat each meal or snack?
- What did you eat at each meal or snack?
- Describe your mind-set during each meal or snack.
- How did you feel after each meal—physically, emotionally, energetically, and mentally?

The awareness developed by doing this assignment in earnest will open your mind and help you to implement the SEAL fuel plan. Contact us if you need some support—we're happy to help you as we helped Michael.

Incidentally, Michael completed the 3-week SEALFIT Academy and Kokoro Camp at age 45. He's now one of our Unbeatable Mind Coaches. He has grown some serious hair on his chest!

YOUR MISSION . . .

WARM-UP: ROM drills, then 20 reps of air squats and push-ups, and 5 dead-hang pull-ups.

WORK CAPACITY: As many rounds as possible (AMRAP) in 20 minutes of:

- 5 pull-ups (substitute band pull-ups or sit-ups if you can't do pull-ups yet)
- 10 push-ups
- 15 air squats. This equals 1 round.

COOL DOWN: 1-mile jog or walk, full body stretch.

COACHING NOTES: Journal your results. Your goal is 15 rounds or more. Full range of motion (ROM) is essential. Five rounds with great ROM is better than 10 rounds of half-assed squats and push-ups. Get your hips below your knees on the air squat, and touch your chest and extend your elbows on the push-ups. Chin over the bar at the top and full extension at bottom of the pull-ups. Attack this workout—try to limit rest to no more than 10 seconds at a time. Feed the courage dog and crush this! DON'T HOLD BACK!

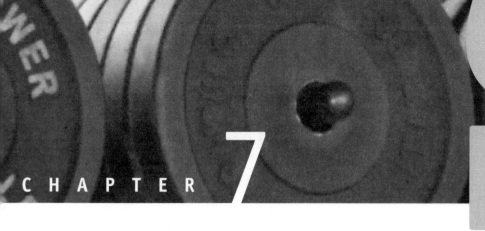

CHAPTER 7

ON-RAMP TRAINING

S EALFIT OFFERS FOUR DISTINCT AND PROGRESSIVE WORKOUT REGIMENS. THIS BOOK BEGINS WITH ON-RAMP TRAINING AND PROCEEDS TO ADVANCED OPERATOR TRAINING. COMPLETE THE ON-RAMP REGIMEN NO MATTER YOUR SKILL OR FITNESS LEVEL. YOU MAY SEE IT AS BENEATH YOU. AS I SAID BEFORE, LOOK AT IT AS A CHANCE TO IMPROVE YOUR BASIC TECHNIQUES. NO PROFESSIONAL ATHLETE EVER REACHES THE LEVEL WHERE HE OR she can skip practicing and improving fundamentals. If you take On-Ramp Training seriously, you'll see breakthroughs in your training performance.

I've included the Basic Training physical workouts as Appendix 2 at the back of the book. If the On-Ramp pushes you to your limits, you may want to substitute the Basic Training workouts for the Advanced Operator Training workouts while still including the rest of the training material. They'll build your total body strength, upper body strength, and lower body strength to prepare them for the increased volume and intensity of the Advanced Operator Training.

If you're a special-ops candidate, explore the Special Operations Candidate Prep template and combine it sensibly with the Advanced Operator Training. The important thing is to adequately assess your level and not take too much on right away. Overtraining is a serious offense that will set you back. Check your ego at the door.

The three primary training sessions have five components:

- Baseline
- Strength
- Stamina
- Work capacity
- Durability

Although section titles are self-explanatory, I'll explain one each week to clear up any questions. If you'd like to know everything in advance, feel free to read ahead. I've included the section on *durability* at the end of the On-Ramp Training chapter, along with our unique SEALFIT Yoga training.

Technique supersedes weight for all strength movements. This also applies to work capacity movements. Remember your ego was checked at the door. The strength movement rep and set scheme is a simple 5 × 5 (5 reps × 5 sets)—first set of 5 will be light, and you will add weight to each additional set until:

- Technique is compromised.
- Failure or the last rep of the last set is near failure.

We'll always come back to fundamentals when performing a barbell movement—stance, grip, and position.

Please scale the movements to your skill level—see Appendix 4 on scaling and substituting exercises. For example, use bands for pull-ups, and do push-ups on your knees as opposed to plank, etc. Thursday will be an active recovery day that works on a long, slow distance. The training week starts on Monday and ends on Friday with Saturday and Sunday as rest days. It's a good idea to walk, practice yoga, swim, or engage in a mild activity on rest days, but don't work too hard.

Durability

When you get to the end of your rope, tie a knot and hang on. —FRANKLIN D. ROOSEVELT

Before you proceed, let's talk about *durability*, your ability to "stay in the game." To become and stay durable, both hard and soft skills are required. You're no good to the team if you get hurt before a mission. Even worse, you're an outright liability if you get hurt during a mission. And if you burn out or lose motivation, you're on the edge of being a liability to yourself *and* the team. Drive home these concepts of durability, followed by SEALFIT Yoga practice, before assaulting the Advanced Operator Training.

Most injuries and accidents arise because the trainee slips into a low state of awareness, becomes fatigued, is ill prepared, or simply screws around. Training durability requires awareness, core engagement, flexibility and mobility, proper fueling and hydration, injury avoidance, and rest.

CORE ENGAGEMENT AND STRENGTH: For SEALFIT purposes, the core is the body's torso. Everything else is referred to as the *extremities*. Core strength is developed with total body exercise that include the overhead squat, squat cleans, and the deadlift. Sandbag work is also particularly effective at developing core strength because of the required rotational work with an unstable load. Fifteen minutes of sandbag get-ups several times a week will develop a rock-solid core. We specifically train for durability during the last segment of SEALFIT. Using core exercises within a cool down ensures that the core doesn't get overlooked. SEALs have a plethora of fun core exercises, so we draw from that goodie bag.

FLEXIBILITY AND MOBILITY: Maybe the most often overlooked aspect of strength training is flexibility and mobility. Range of motion is critical to maintaining durability over the long haul.

INJURY AVOIDANCE: "Proper prior preparation prevents piss-poor performance" is the SEAL mantra for initially taking extra time to ensure that you don't eat it later. Take time to prepare your feet for a long ruck or your hands for a 100 pull-up workout to prevent nasty and nagging injuries. Blisters and torn calluses hamper performance and slow your team down. Active warm-up and ROM drills prior to a workout will help avoid shock injuries like pulled hamstrings.

HYDRATION AND REFUELING: Drink lots of fresh water and use electrolytes to avoid cramping. Generally, drink half your body weight in ounces of water throughout the day. Drink liberally before, during, and after a training session. Refuel with a protein-laden snack within 30 minutes of a session. For sessions longer than an hour, snack during the workout. Hydrating and refueling must become a discipline. Sporadically remembering to hydrate means that you're dehydrated. Dehydration and undernourishment will lead to a declining performance, low motivation, and possible injury.

REST AND RECOVERY: As important as hydration and refueling, program rest and recovery into your training regimen. Encourage your team to take training time-outs, or days off, when they feel depleted. Get 8 hours of good, restful sleep a night. It's not always practical for SEAL operators, but for everyone else, do it. Growth hormones release only when you're in REM sleep, which is the third cycle of sleep. Avoid sugar, including alcohol, prior to bedtime, because sugar inhibits sleep patterns and hinders muscle recovery and growth.

SEALFIT Yoga Forms

SEALFIT Yoga utilizes a variety of poses sequenced by the objectives of each training session. The session may be a recovery or a hard session. Primary poses include:

- **BALANCING:** Predominantly standing poses that develop balance in our minds and bodies.

- **STRENGTHENING:** Core poses that focus or rely on arm balance. These are typically the most challenging.

- **LENGTHENING AND EXTENDING:** Poses most commonly associated with yoga, which have been used as stretching exercises in athletic training for years.

- **RESTORING AND CONTRACTING:** Poses that help lengthen your spinal column and are closely related to lengthening poses. For every lengthening pose there is a contracting pose.

- ■ CLEANSING: Poses that typically show up as twists. The twists compress and "wring out" your internal organs.

- ■ INVERSION: Poses that include the plow, headstand, handstand, shoulder stand, and variations for each. In these poses, the blood flows in the opposite direction from normal and the organs "hang" upside down. It's very healthy for your body.

- ■ RESTING: Poses that are used as finishing poses. Examples include *shavasana* (the dead man's pose) that ends every practice.

SEALFIT Yoga Body Awareness and Control

SEALFIT Yoga brings deep awareness in understanding how the body moves and works. Senses are turned inward to "listen and feel" with refined skills. This practice deepens your intuition. Awareness spills into physical fitness training to help you move with purpose and sensitivity to the quality of movement. This eventually leads to virtuosity.

CORE DEVELOPMENT: Yoga and its core strength are built at a very deep root level. Core strength leads to the seemingly magical powers of arm balances and poses whereby trainees can hover a foot off the floor by balancing on their palms. Core strength supplements the core development that occurs through functional strength training.

CONCENTRATION DEVELOPMENT: A primary benefit and focus of yoga practice is to deepen your concentration. SEALFIT Yoga is moving concentration practice that includes seated concentration between breath control and visualization.

BALANCE: Balance starts with a calm mind and extends to your core grounding itself with the earth. Balance in yoga is more subtle than typical athletic balance and can lead you to be more graceful in your physical endeavors.

FLOW: Yoga movements flow from one to another such that the practice has qualities like a dance, or kata. This flow stokes internal heat and allows you to link movements to your breathing.

ENERGY MOVEMENT: Moving your internal energy (prana, ki, force) intentionally is the focus of the breathing practices and occurs as part of the flow of your yoga practice. This provides many health benefits and allows you to muster this internal energy and forcefully project it.

DETOXIFYING: Twisting and bending mash your internal organs like a washing machine and lead to internal organ detoxification and cleansing.

INCREASED PRESENCE: The intense concentration required of SEALFIT Yoga can lead to moments of complete release when your mind is devoid of thought and you're fully focused on the present moment. Finding this state while moving in yoga helps you to transfer this esoteric skill to the arena of fitness training and life. You can then find more calm and focused attention in the chaos of a workout, or life in general.

Short Form A (see www.sealfit.com/yoga)

- 5x Sun Salutation A, hold down dogs for 5 breaths
- transition breathing exercises
- windmill
- flow to seated poses
- forward bend—flow
- table top—flow
- twist 1
- box breathing 5 cycles
- dead man's pose

Short Form B (see www.sealfit.com/yoga)

- 3x Sun Salutation A, hold down dogs for 5 breaths
- 3x Sun Salutation B, hold down dogs for 5 breaths
- transition breathing exercises
- windmill
- flow to seated poses

- forward bend—flow
- table top—flow
- twist 1
- box breathing 5 cycles
- dead man's pose

Hip Mobility Drill (see www.sealfit.com/yoga)

- Samson Stretch—right leg back
- inside twist
- outside twist
- pigeon
- plank
- upward-facing dog to downward-facing dog
- Samson Stretch—left leg back
- inside twist
- outside twist
- pigeon
- plank
- upward-facing dog to downward-facing dog
- third world squat
- standing forward bend

Shoulder Mobility Drill (with PVC or broomstick) (see www.sealfit.com/yoga)

- neck and shoulder rotations
- 5x PVC shoulder push-pull and passovers
- 3x PVC Figure 8s, each side

- 1x PVC shoulder opener, each side

- 1x PVC behind-the-back forward bend

- 10x overhead squats

- inside-outside twist with PVC, both sides

Congratulations on completing your first week of SEALFIT training—stand by for a heck of a lot more fun!

SUN SALUTATION A

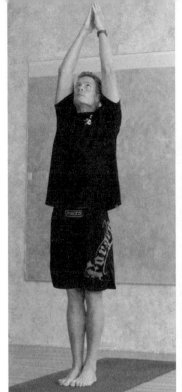

A1

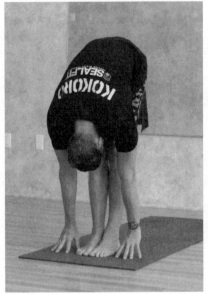

A2

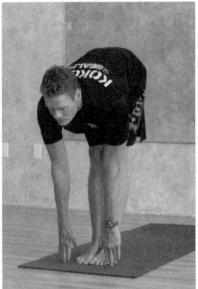

A3

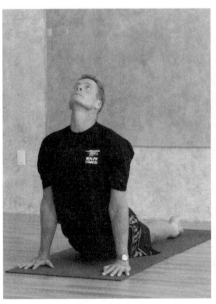

A6

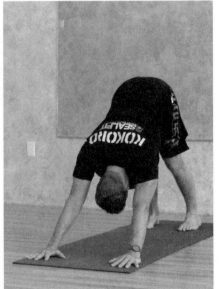

A7

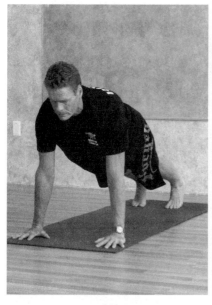

A4

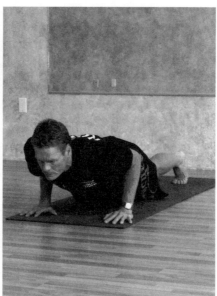

A5

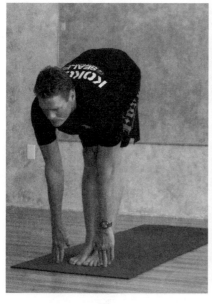

A8

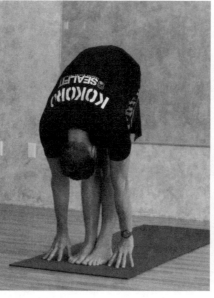

A9

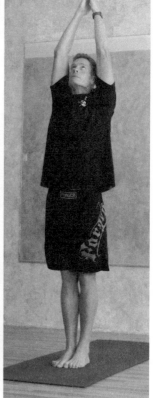

A10

SUN SALUTATION B

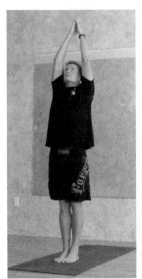

B1

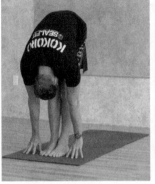

B2

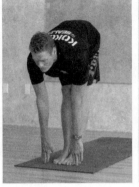

B3

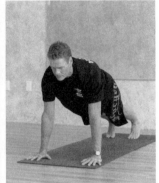

B4

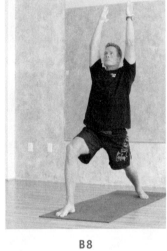

B8

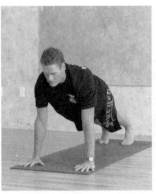

B9

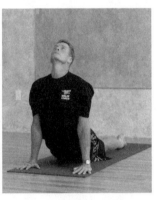

B10

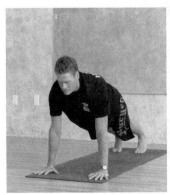

B13

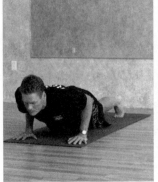

B14

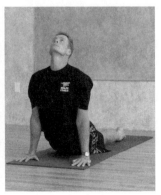

B15

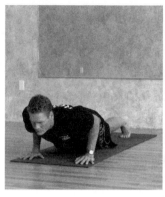

B5

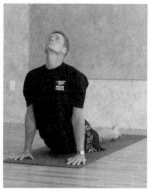

B6

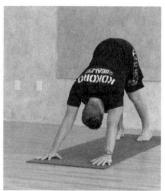

B7

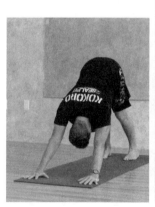

B11

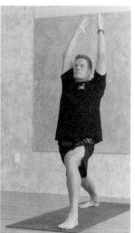

B12

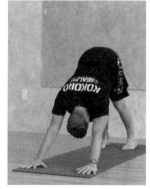

B16

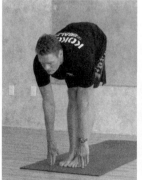

B17

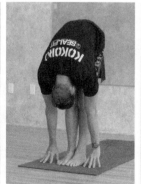

B18

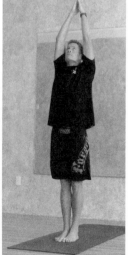

B19

Week 1: The Baseline

Each training session starts with a baseline that's more than a warm-up. The *baseline* is a prep phase used to welcome new trainees, brief the training session, answer questions about the protocol, and demonstrate proper form, function, and posture. I like to begin with a box breathing exercise followed by a series of ROM drills (see www.sealfit.com/videos) and a short run and body blast/row. On strength-training days SEALFIT warms up to the weights that will be used. If it's not a *strength* day, SEALFIT prepares for the *work capacity* or *endurance* section. *Baseline* is named as such because the system baselines all trainees in the reality of the moment to prepare for what's ahead.

Remember, a SEALFIT training session is not a workout. We don't just saunter into the gym and start the SEALFIT workout. SEALFIT is treated with a degree of importance that doesn't ignore important details. SEALFIT is most often done with a team. The team will start on time, have a working plan, and have a brief/debrief of each session. I like to practice the Five Mountains during each training session and look for opportunities to train mental toughness, emotional control, and the warrior spirit. These opportunities are not hard to discover during the training sessions for a good coach. The more energy you put into the seriousness of the training session, as you maintain focus, intensity, and a sense of teamwork, the more you'll get out of each session.

WEEK 1, NEW MOVEMENTS: row, sit-up, pull-up, back squat, knees to elbows, front squat, overhead squat, and step-ups.

NOTE: Please see Appendix 5 for a list of acronyms and abbreviations.

Discipline

There once was a strong and self-confident young man who dreamed of greatness. One day, after watching *Zero Dark Thirty,* his friend told him of a man in California who could virtually guarantee him a coveted SEAL position. His eyes glowed. As long as he could remember, he'd desired this prize. Ultimate manhood and recognition awaited!

He strapped on his knapsack and began a long trek to find out if the legend was real. Challenges lay in store. Mountains stood in his path. But the young man was strong. He wouldn't wait any longer than necessary. He stuck to the highway, impatient and hungry. He hurried his pace. Finally he located the wise man and made his appearance.

"I want to learn all I can from you and earn the Navy SEAL Trident!"

"I see," the wise old man said kindly. "Drink some tea. We'll talk about it further."

The old man turned on his teapot and sat quietly, waiting for the water to boil. The young man squirmed in his seat. Unable to wait any longer, he lit in.

"What do you recommend I do? Someone told me I should run forty miles a week. What fins should I use? How do I improve my pull-ups? I'm only at fifteen . . ."

The teapot started to sing. The wise man said nothing as the young man prattled on. He picked up the pot and began to pour. Tea reached the top of the cup, yet he kept pouring. He smiled kindly as it spilled onto the table. Then it reached the visitor's lap. The young guy said nothing at first, wondering if the old man was senile or something.

"Sir, stop pouring. The tea's going all over the place!"

"Yes it is, isn't it? Interesting. Just like your mind, it's running all over the place."

The young man grew angry as the old man continued.

"Your mind is so full of ideas . . . how strong and athletic you are . . . this tip . . . that trick. There's no room left for me to help you. Please. Empty your cup. Come back when you're ready to learn."

What kind of game was this guy playing? thought the young man. His emotions spun from anger to frustration to dejection. Everything had come easy to him in life, and here was some nut telling him to empty his cup. *What the hell?* He stormed off, resolved to become a SEAL on his own.

Nine months later, Day 2 of Hell Week, the young man's body lay broken. He could barely lift his arms. His mind was weary. He tried to dig deep within for more strength and stamina. It wasn't enough. His helmet came to rest beside the other dropouts in a solemn line of defeat.

I SEE THIS ALL THE time. It's a busy world. You have many commitments. But discipline requires that you learn a new way of thinking and acting, one where you control your mind and emotions first. Is your cup running over? Do you struggle to find time and energy to train? Is your mind running about and constantly obsessing about this supplement or that, this new training tool or that?

The biblical concept of tithing has you pay God first, then yourself, then the merchant, and then the tax man. Try it for growth—discipline yourself to spend the first 10 percent of your day on your mental, emotional, and spiritual training. Empty your cup to learn. Fill it with far more value to give to the world. Now let's get to work!

MONDAY

BASELINE: presession SOP and box breathing for 5 minutes. Box breathing.

- ROM drills
- 3 rounds—200m run, 10x air squats, 10x arm circles (10 forward and 10 back)

STRENGTH: back squat (www.sealfit.com/videos)—5 reps × 5 sets. Keep the load light (45# bar to 95#).

WORK CAPACITY: baseline for time completed:

- 500m row (if you do not have a rower, substitute a run)
- 40x air squats
- 30x sit-ups
- 20x push-ups
- 10x pull-ups (if you're unable to perform a pull-up, perform jumping pull-ups or use a band)

DURABILITY: SEALFIT Yoga hip and shoulder mobility drills. Hydrate and fuel within 30 minutes. Journal post-training session SOP.

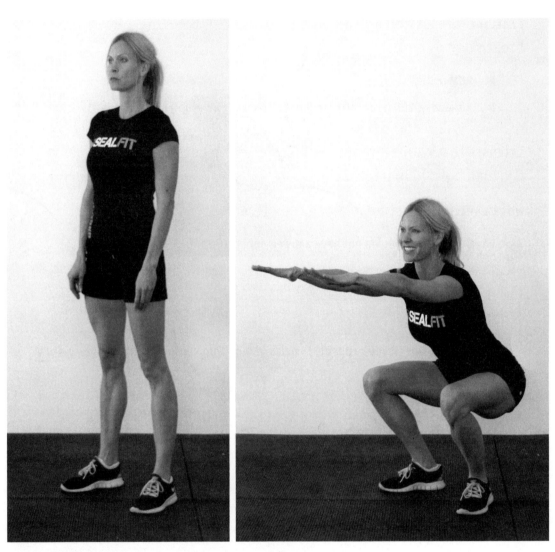

AIR SQUATS

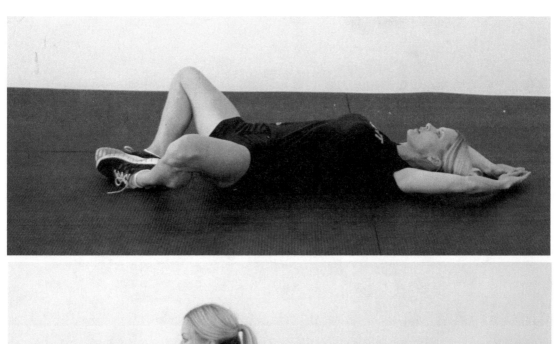

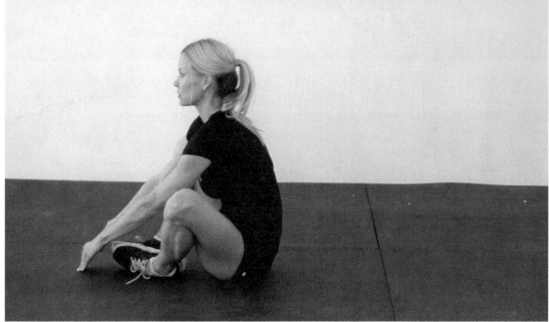

SIT-UPS

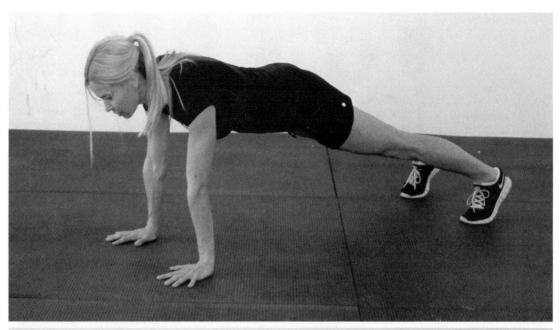

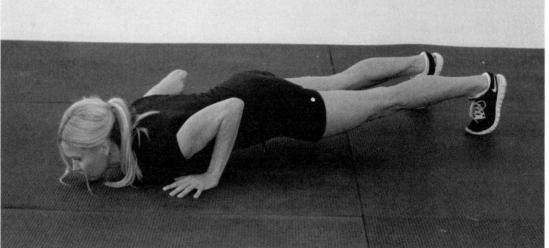

PUSH-UPS

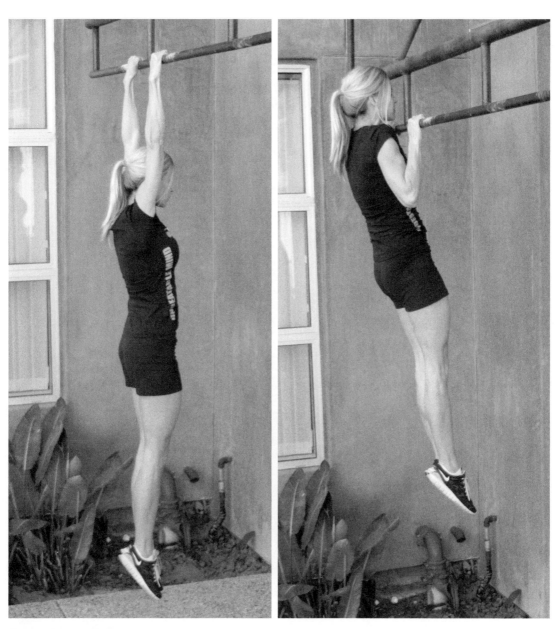

PULL-UPS

TUESDAY [WEEK 1: THE BASELINE]

BASELINE: pre-SOP and box breathing

- ROM drills
- 200m run
- 20x 2-count mountain climbers
- 200m run
- 20 push-ups

WORK CAPACITY: complete 3 RFT of:

- 400m run
- 10x burpees
- 10x back squats (45#/35#)
- 10x knees to elbow

DURABILITY: SEALFIT Yoga Short Form A or active stretch. Hydrate and fuel within 30 minutes. Journal post-training session SOP.

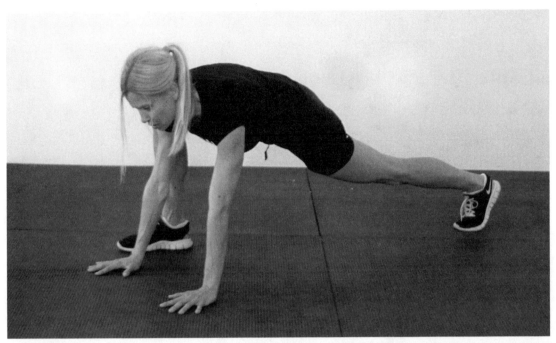

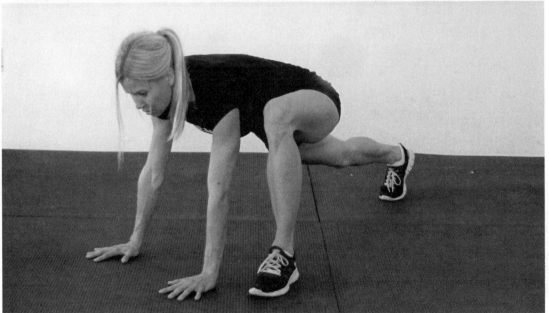

MOUNTAIN CLIMBERS

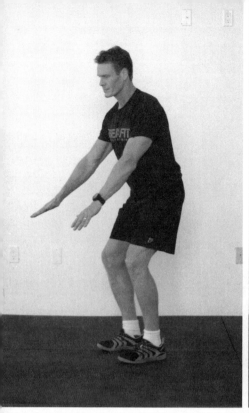

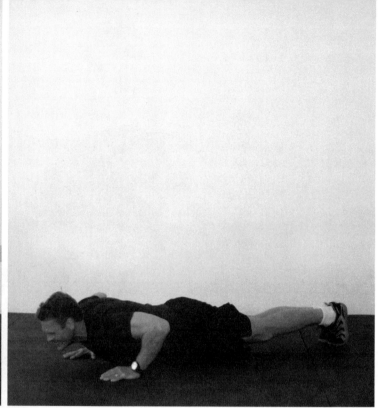

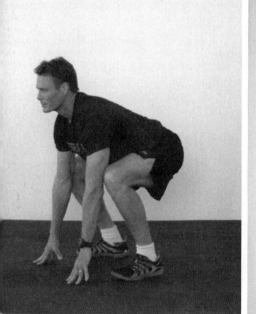

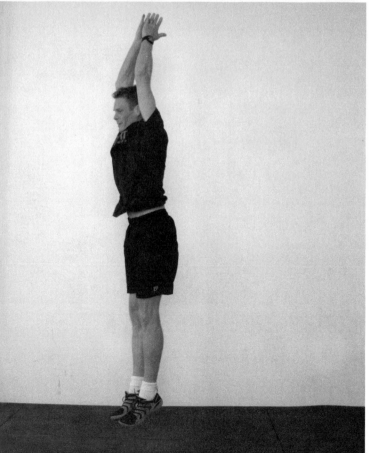

BURPEES

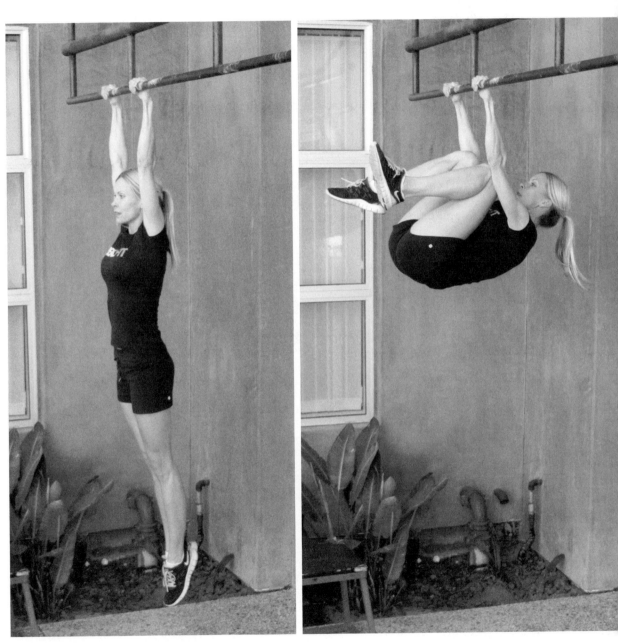

KNEES TO ELBOWS

WEDNESDAY [WEEK 1: THE BASELINE]

BASELINE: pre-SOP and box breathing

- ROM drills
- 400m run
- 5 rounds—5x air squats, 5x back squats (barbell), 5x push-ups, 5x sit-ups

STRENGTH: front squat (www.sealfit.com/videos)—5 reps × 5 sets

WORK CAPACITY: complete AMRAP in 10 minutes:

- 5x pull-ups (scale as needed)
- 7x push-ups
- 9x front squats (45#/35#)

DURABILITY: SEALFIT Yoga Short Form B or active stretch. Hydrate and fuel within 30 minutes. Journal post-training session SOP.

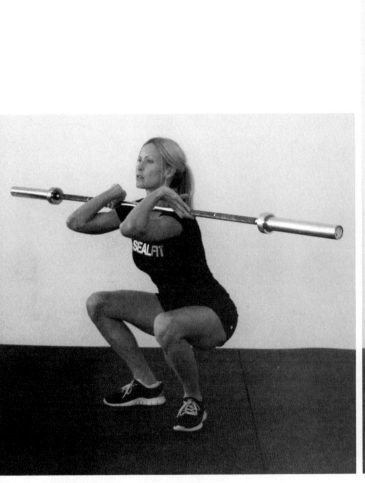
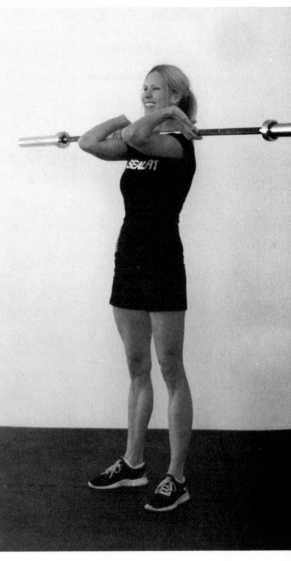

FRONT SQUATS

THURSDAY [WEEK 1: THE BASELINE]

BASELINE: pre-SOP and box breathing

- ROM drills
- 20 minutes of grinder PT (www.sealfit.com/videos)

ENDURANCE: 10 minutes of LSD run, ruck, or swim

DURABILITY: SEALFIT Yoga or active stretch. Hydrate and fuel within 30 minutes. Journal post-training session SOP.

BASELINE: pre-SOP and box breathing

- ROM drills
- 3 rounds—150m row, 10x air squats, 10x front squats (barbell)

STRENGTH: overhead squat (www.sealfit.com/videos)—5 reps × 5 sets

WORK CAPACITY: complete 10–9–8–7–6–5–4–3–2–1 (10 reps of each exercise followed by 9 reps of each exercise, etc.) of:

- overhead squat (barbell, light barbell, or PVC pipe)
- step-ups each leg (15-inch box)
- sit-ups

DURABILITY: SEALFIT Yoga Short Form A or active stretch. Hydrate and fuel within 30 minutes. Journal post-training session SOP.

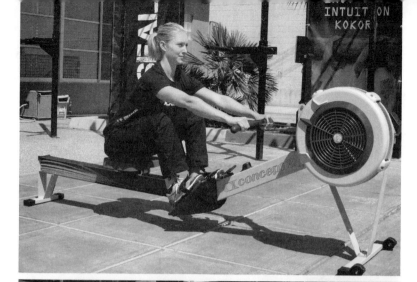

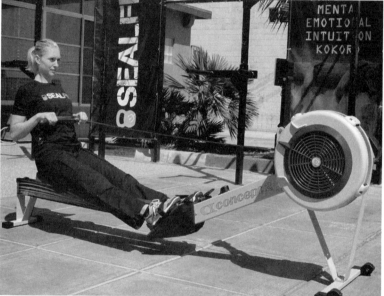

ROWS

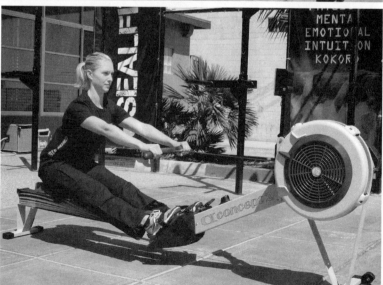

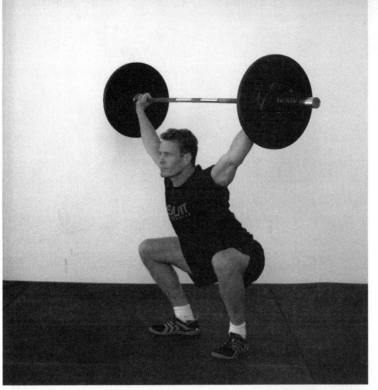

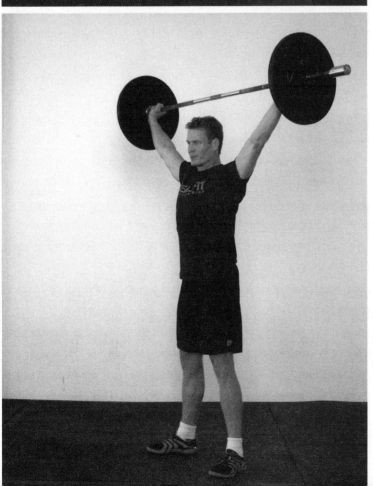

OVERHEAD SQUATS

Week 2: Strength

SEALFIT strength training is 4 days a week that includes (with some exception) lower (*back squat*), upper (*push press*), and total body lifts (*deadlift* and *bench press*). The overhead squat, weighted pull-ups, and front squat are occasionally cycled in. Narrowing the strength lifts to the four listed above leads to more focused results. If you would like additional reading on strength training, I recommend Mark Rippetoe's *Starting Strength* as a great resource for beginning lifters. There are great exercise videos on the SEALFIT YouTube channel as well.

New trainees must stay focused on their form and use lighter loads until strength-training lifts are safely performed. All egos must be in check. Injury will occur if you move too fast or try to impress your girlfriend and teammates. Deadlifts and back squats take time to develop core strength and the necessary lower lumbar stability that protects the spine during the execution of the movement.

Evidence suggests that tall endurance athletes—like me—are keenly at risk with the execution of the deadlift and the back squat. I've injured my back twice executing each lift during my early years by going too far, too fast. Tall recovering triathletes will never lift as much as a shorter powerlifter. And a former powerlifter will never run as fast or far as a former triathlete, so we're even! So, if you're a tall endurance athlete, consider performing a deadlift elevated off the ground with a 45-pound plate under each side. There's no reason to go for a 1 Round Max effort every time you lift. You'll make more gains by sticking with 10, 5, and 3 Round Max efforts. My injuries have all occurred during 1 Round Max attempts. Once I learned how to train properly, my injuries stopped. And I've been injury free for years . . . knock on wood.

Quite simply, strength increases your durability and ability to carry heavy loads, which makes you more useful to your team.

We chose the four primary lifts for their simplicity, their functionality, and their ability to convey strength gains across the body's entire system. These lifts also allow you to lift heavy loads. Lifting heavy loads helps to develop your confidence and courage. There's also growing evidence that your neuroendocrine system is stimulated to release growth hormones when lifting your body weight or an even greater load, which is achievable with each of the four lifts.

Advance Operator Training cycles strength training in order to develop strength, stamina, raw strength, strength power, and finally a personal best strength max load. A de-load week occurs prior to the personal best week to give your mind and body a much-needed break.

During the baseline, you'll work to gain a max working load by starting with a light load and high rep scheme and progressively increasing the load while reducing reps until you reach or are near to a 1 rep max. This effort should take 10 to 15 minutes.

You'll start the actual strength session when you (and your team) are happy with your warm-up and you're executing your working load. You'll follow a prescribed protocol—a set number of sets and reps at −5 percent or −10 percent of the max load. This submaximal work is designed to "push the envelope" and condition your body and mind to work at loads near your max. The number of sets and reps vary for each phase.

Strength training is never timed or completed with expediency. At SEALFIT HQ, we train for strength in an alert, methodical, yet casual manner. You don't want to be tense during strength training. It's important to maintain a relaxed focus and be aware of what's going on in and around you as you maintain a safe training environment. At the same time, you can chat, share ideas, work on form, correct a teammate's form, joke, and generally build the team's morale.

WEEK 2, NEW MOVEMENTS: strict press, supine ring pull-up, walking lunge, push press, ball slam, push jerk.

Overhead press strength-training movements:

- strict press
- push press
- push jerk

The start and end position for each movement is the same. How the weight is raised overhead is the only difference.

Perform a **strict press** as the barbell rests on your shoulders without holding any weight in your arms. This requires elements of mobility. You grip the barbell directly in the hands—not back on the fingertips, like you hold the barbell for the front squat. Point your elbows down. From this position, press the barbell overhead until the weight is secured and held slightly behind your ears. Keep your legs locked straight and your glutes, core, and hamstrings tight.

Add a dip-drive for the **push press** and use your legs to help push the bar overhead. This piston-like, down-up explosive movement literally throws the bar off your chest. Finish the motion by pressing your arms the same way you would during a strict press. Typically you can push-press 30 percent more load overhead. The push press is a much more functional movement than the strict press, although it doesn't gauge raw strength as well as the strict press. Coaching cues for the dip include bending at the knees and not the waist and taking a deep breath prior to the dip-drive—don't inhale as you dip. Drive up with your legs and at the last minute engage the arms to finish the movement. Dip, drive, and press!!!

The **push jerk** is a quick, aggressive movement more so than both the strict press and push press. It focuses on jumping your body underneath the bar, instead up pushing it up with your arms. As you dip and drive the bar up and off your shoulders, jump your body down under the bar so that you receive the weight locked out overhead in one motion. This Olympic lift also known as the "jerk" in the *clean and jerk* can be awkward for beginners. Work on the execution simulating a PVC pipe for a barbell to get the hang of it. Watch the videos (www.sealfit.com/videos), or better yet, hire a coach to work on the "Oly" lifts with you. You'll be able to push-jerk at least 30 percent more than the push press, assuming that your form is legitimate.

Integrity

"Lieutenant Divine, I need to speak with you, sir." Johnson peeked nervously through the door into the Alpha Platoon space.

"What's up?" I said, busy preparing for our pending deployment to Iraq for Desert Shield.

"Well, sir, you see, ah . . ."

"Spit it out, Johnson. I have a lot to do to get ready, and so do you."

"I'm not going!"

"What do you mean, exactly? . . . You're not going where?"

"I'm not going to Iraq." He gave me a strange look.

At first I didn't believe him, but the look on his face . . . It made me feel squeamish. This had never happened in the SEALs before.

"I'm a conscientious objector."

"What the F! Are you serious? After all that work to get into BUD/S, make it through training, a year work-up with Alpha Platoon, and you're not going to deploy???

"Johnson, do you know what integrity is? It's when you do what you say and say what you think. You just put Alpha Platoon through a twelve-month integrity breach. All this time you knew we'd probably go to war. Now on the cusp of jumping off the ramp, you're bailing."

The look disappeared from his face. His eyes found the floor. Here was a Trident wearer who'd gone into the SEALs just to see if he could make it, with no intention of ever actually doing the job. He never could look me in the eye again. What a waste.

Integrity breaches don't have to be this blatant to corrode your character or your team's trust. I'm sure you've met many "smiling screws" who play nice and then stab you in the back. That's what Johnson did to his team.

We all have weak spots. Take a moment to look for any integrity breaches in your own life. Note them in your journal and your specific plan to change them. It's time to be honest in all your actions, big and small. Pay attention to your thoughts. Speak only words of truth that are also helpful and positive. Otherwise, remain silent. Let your actions speak your character.

Now stay safe, remain focused, and have fun!

MONDAY

BASELINE: pre-SOP and box breathing

- ROM drills
- 30–20–10 reps of jumping jacks, air squats, and arm circles

STRENGTH: strict press (www.sealfit.com/videos)—5 reps × 5 sets

WORK CAPACITY: complete the following for time:

- 1,000m row
- 25x strict presses (45#/35#)
- 20x supine ring pull-ups

DURABILITY: SEALFIT Yoga shoulder mobility drill or active stretch. Hydrate and fuel within 30 minutes. Journal post-training session SOP.

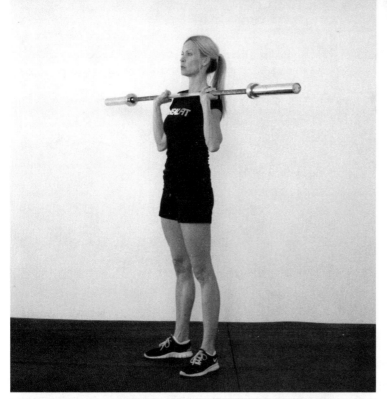

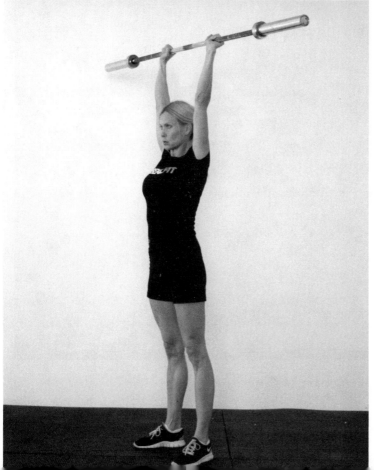

STRICT
PRESSES

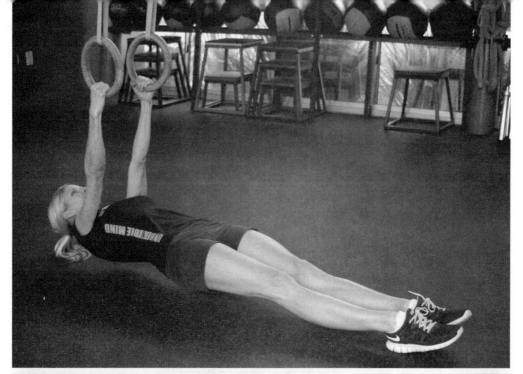

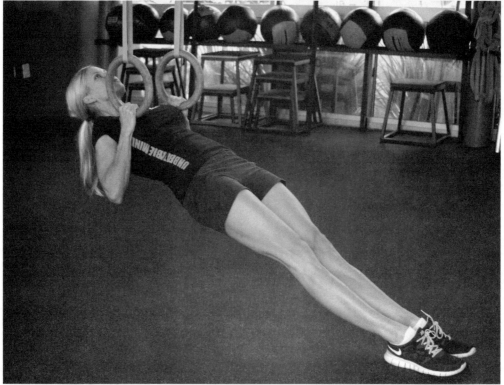

SUPINE RING PULL-UPS

BASELINE: pre-SOP and box breathing

- ROM drills
- 500m run
- 3 rounds—5x walking lunges each leg, 10x push-ups, 15x sit-ups

WORK CAPACITY: AMRAP in 20 minutes:

- 25m walking lunge
- 10x burpees
- 25m jog back to starting point

DURABILITY: SEALFIT Yoga hip mobility drill or active stretch. Hydrate and fuel within 30 minutes. Journal post-training session SOP.

WEDNESDAY [WEEK 2: STRENGTH]

BASELINE: pre-SOP and box breathing

- ROM drills
- 3 rounds—200m run, 5x strict presses (45#/35#), 5x dips, 5x jumping squats

STRENGTH: push press (www.sealfit.com/videos)—5 reps × 5 sets

WORK CAPACITY: complete 4 RFT of:

- 400m run
- 10x push presses (45#)
- 10x ball slams (20#/12#)

DURABILITY: SEALFIT Yoga Short Form A or active stretch. Hydrate and fuel within 30 minutes. Journal post-training session SOP.

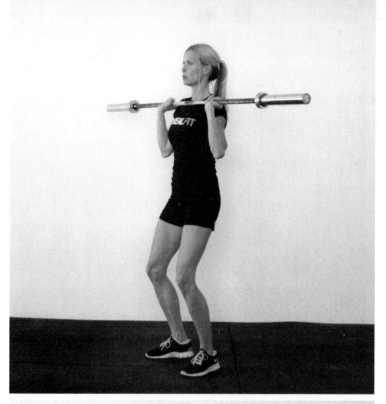

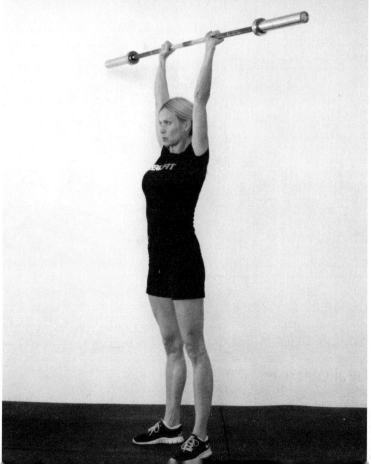

PUSH PRESSES

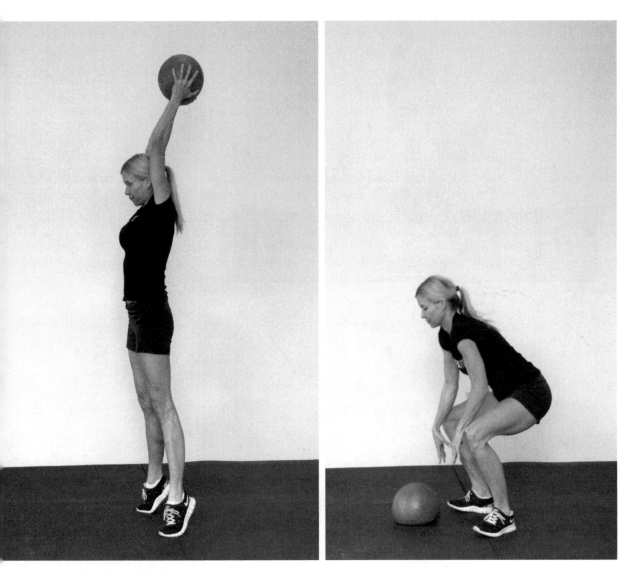

BALL SLAMS

BASELINE: pre-SOP and box breathing

- ROM drills
- 20 minutes of grinder PT

ENDURANCE: 15 minutes of LSD run, ruck, or swim

DURABILITY: SEALFIT Yoga (any form) or active stretch. Hydrate and fuel within 30 minutes. Journal post-training session SOP.

FRIDAY [WEEK 2: STRENGTH]

BASELINE: pre-SOP and box breathing

- ROM drills
- 250m row, 15x push-ups
- 250m row, 15x push presses (45#/35#)

STRENGTH: push jerk (www.sealfit.com/videos)—5 reps × 5 sets

WORK CAPACITY: complete 21–15–9 reps for time (21 reps of each exercise, followed by 15 reps of each exercise, and then 9):

- 4-count mountain climbers
- push jerk (45#/35#)
- sit-ups

DURABILITY: SEALFIT Yoga Short Form B or active stretch. Hydrate and fuel within 30 minutes. Journal post-training session SOP.

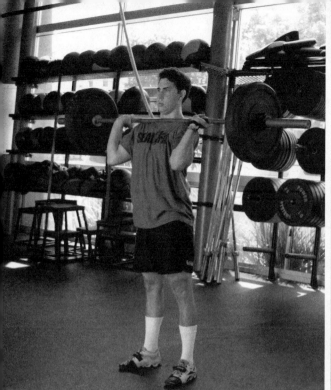
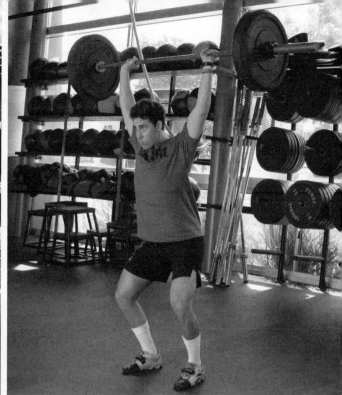
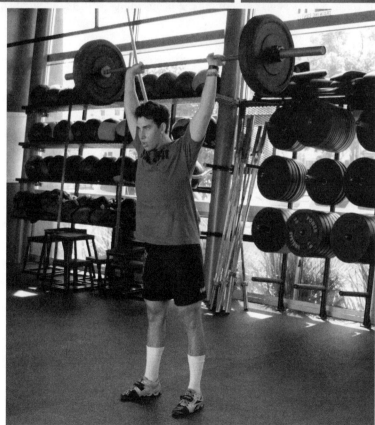

PUSH JERKS

Week 3: Stamina

The stamina section increases intensity and pace, but it's not timed or considered high-intensity interval training. I characterize stamina as moderate intensity, volume training, with two primary models.

1. The *chipper* will "chip" through a large number of reps for each exercise before moving on to the next. For example, 50 deadlifts at 40 percent max load, followed by 75 box jumps, finishing with an 800m buddy carry.

2. The RFC (rounds done for completion) is not timed. For example, complete 4 rounds of 12x deadlifts at 40 percent max, 20x box jumps, and a 50m buddy pull with a heavy band.

I love the strength and stamina phase of a workout. It's both challenging and fun because the pressure of time is no longer a factor. But in case you let your guard down, stand by. *Work capacity* is next!

WEEK 3, NEW MOVEMENTS: DB push press, deadlift, thruster, sumo deadlift high pull, wall ball, dips, power clean.

I cannot state emphatically enough the importance of proper technique while performing each lift. Remember the basic fundamentals of stance, grip, and position.

The proper starting position for the **deadlift** begins with your feet under your hips—known as the pulling position. Grip the bar one thumb length from the smooth part of the bar, on the outside of the knurling. Keep your butt down, chest up, and arch your lower back. Push the ground away from you rather than pulling with your arms at the start of the lift. Avoid the "grip and rip" syndrome. Rather, seek a "smooth" push away from the floor before accelerating with your hips open. Maintain your weight in your heels and keep the bar as close to your shins as possible. Most important—lift with your legs, not your back!

The **power clean** starts exactly the same way as the deadlift. However, once the bar moves above your knees, you'll jump the barbell up to your shoulders in the front squat rack position. The Burgener Warm-up named after Coach Mike Burgener is a great tool for learning Olympic lifts. I highly recommend that you watch the video (www.sealfit.com /videos) before progressing on the lifts.

Trust Your Gut

> When you burn your boats with full-in commitment, you elevate risk and remove the safety net. This mobilizes the team to violently focus on mission accomplishment. But there's no turning back—you must be 100 percent confident in this decision. All of your skills and instincts come to bear on that one moment of choice. Then you just go for it. If things don't go according to plan, and they won't . . . you have no choice but to find a way to the other side.

A memory popped into my head as I spoke those words to the academy class. It had occurred right before I left SEAL Team 3 for a new assignment.

THE WEATHER WAS ROUGH, THE surf massive. Alpha Platoon stood ready to deploy for combat. Only an operational readiness test, and the weather, remained for them to conquer. Their mission: a direct action inserting at Morro Bay on the Northern California coast—via rigid-hulled inflatable boats (RHIBs). Navigating the RHIBs to the insertion point, Lieutenant Englehart, the new platoon commander, sent in his swimmer scouts to check things out. It looked risky, and his team was eager. Having the team's commanding officer (CO) in the boat increased his anxiety.

"I don't know, Lieutenant," said Brown, the lead scout, surfacing near the boats. "I made it to the outer zone. Waves cresting near twenty feet and coming in fast. It's sketchy."

He wanted this exam to go smoothly. The CO wanted to push the envelope. The weather pushed them on its edge. His gut felt tight, almost knotted. Images of scattered bodies flashed in his head. "What do you think, Brown?"

Brown scanned the horizon, sniffing the air. "I say no go."

The CO made his way over. The lieutenant hung in an awkward position. This was his platoon and his test, but the CO was the senior officer. He wasn't sure of the RHIBs' capabilities in this size surf. The CO wanted to go for it. The consequences as senior officer on site fell to the CO if it went to shit.

"Let's do this," the lieutenant said. The expert navigators put their noses to the surf, waiting for a lull. *There!* The massive engines roared. Two boats, with sixteen SEALs, bolted toward their destiny. No turning back. Operators perched on toes, muscles taut and eager. Two boats sped side by side into an approaching wave. Higher and higher it crested. A rogue wave! The timing was perfectly wrong.

The lieutenant and the CO glanced at each other with an "Oh, shit" look.

"Hang on!"

Both boats flew ass over teakettle, landing upside down. Operators bobbed in the sea like flotsam, a few knocked unconscious. Instantly they mobilized, hauling injured men onto anything that floated. The SEALs eventually made it to the beach. The mission went on.

"I'm never ignoring my gut again," the lieutenant said to Brown as he motioned his men to move out.

LEARN TO TRUST YOUR GUT. Pay close attention to the feelings and images that churn your stomach or whisper unease. They could change the course of your life.

Heighten your awareness as you train. Look for gut *signals* as you work on the breathing and meditation skills. They're an intuition game changer. They'll free you to commit 100 percent, instead of something less, like the lieutenant did.

As always, train hard, stay safe, and have fun!

BASELINE: pre-SOP and box breathing

- ROM drills
- 400m run
- 10–8–6–4–2 reps of air squats, jumping pull-ups

STRENGTH: deadlift (www.sealfit.com/videos)—5 reps × 5 sets

WORK CAPACITY: complete 5 RFT of:

- 3x deadlifts (95#/65#)
- 6x DB (dumbbell) push presses (25#/15#)
- 9x burpees

DURABILITY: SEALFIT Yoga Short Form A or active stretch. Hydrate and fuel within 30 minutes. Journal post-training session SOP.

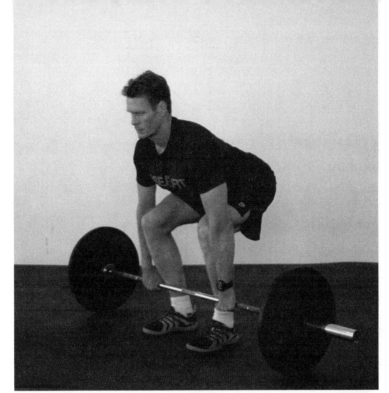

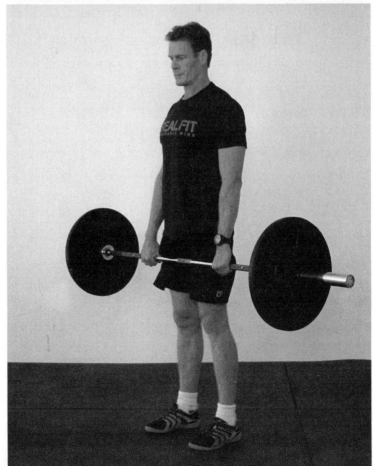

DEADLIFTS

BASELINE: pre-SOP and box breathing

- ROM drills
- 3 rounds—200m run, 25x jumping jacks, 15x sit-ups, 5x hand release push-ups

WORK CAPACITY: complete AMRAP in 20 minutes:

- 400m run
- 10x thruster (www.sealfit.com/videos) (45#/35#)
- 10x knees to elbows

DURABILITY: SEALFIT Yoga hip mobility drill or active stretch. Hydrate and fuel within 30 minutes. Journal post-training session SOP.

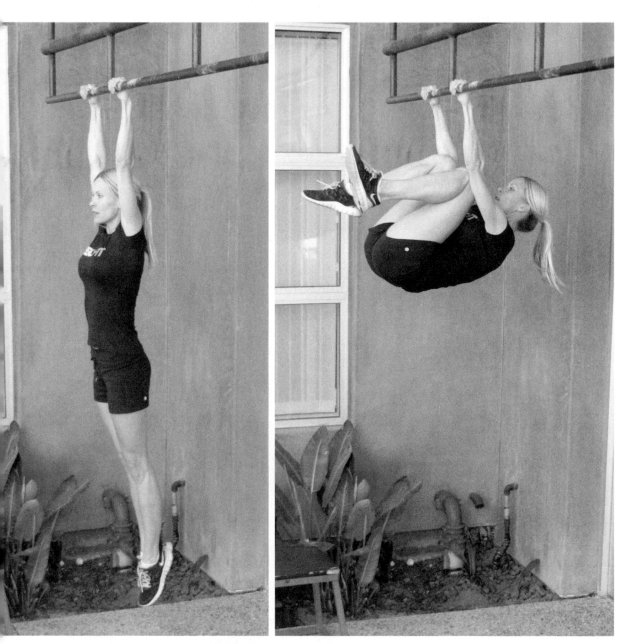

KNEES TO ELBOWS

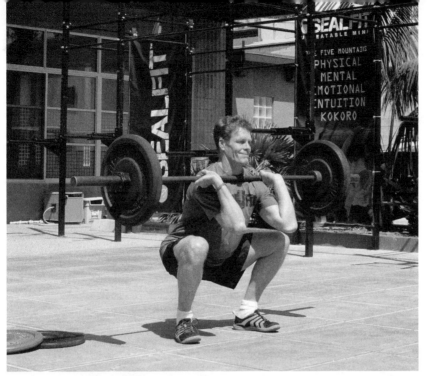

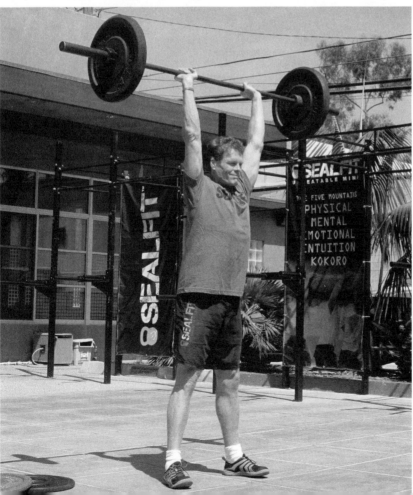

THRUSTERS

WEDNESDAY [WEEK 3: STAMINA]

BASELINE: pre-SOP and box breathing

- ROM drills
- 500m row
- 3 rounds—10x KB deadlifts (16kg/12kg), 10x 2-count mountain climbers, 10x push jerks (45#/35#)

STRENGTH: SDHP (sumo deadlift high pull) (www.sealfit.com/videos) —5 reps × 5 sets

WORK CAPACITY: complete the following for time:

- 500m row
- 25x SDHP (65#/45#)
- 25x wall balls (14#/8#)
- 25x dips
- 500m row

DURABILITY: SEALFIT Yoga Short Form B or active stretch. Hydrate and fuel within 30 minutes. Journal post-training session SOP.

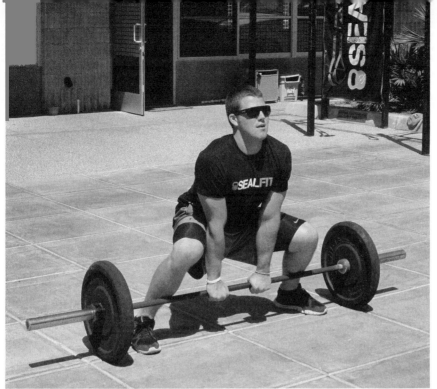

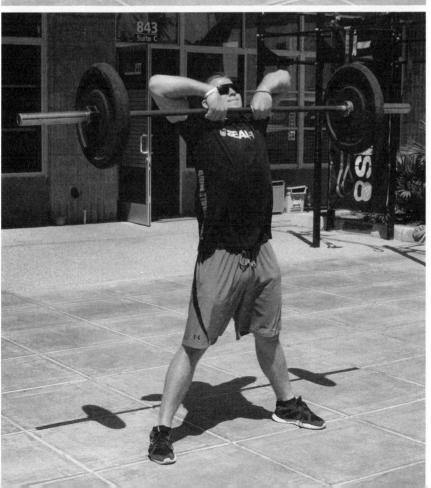

SDHPs

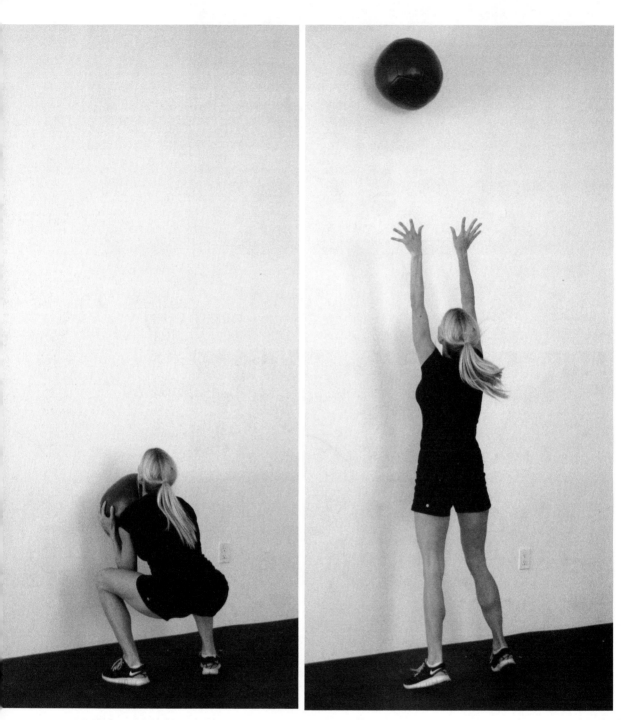

WALL BALLS

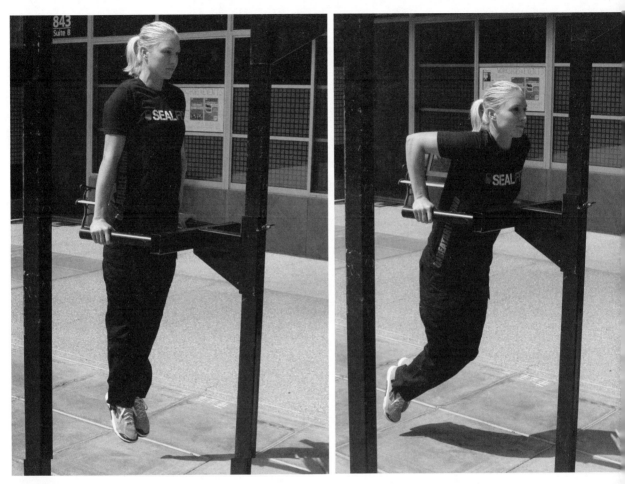

DIPS

THURSDAY [WEEK 3: STAMINA]

BASELINE:

- ROM drills
- 20 minutes of grinder PT

ENDURANCE: 20 minutes of LSD run, ruck, or swim

DURABILITY: SEALFIT Yoga (any form) or active stretch. Hydrate and fuel within 30 minutes. Journal post-training session SOP.

BASELINE: pre-SOP and box breathing

- ROM drills
- 10x sandbag cleans left side (40#/30#)
- 400m run
- 10x sandbag cleans right side (40#/30#)
- Burgener Warm-up—clean grip

STRENGTH: power clean—5 reps × 5 sets

WORK CAPACITY: complete 5 rounds of the following:

- 10x power cleans (95#/65#)
- 100m run
- 30-second rest

DURABILITY: SEALFIT Yoga shoulder mobility drill or active stretch. Hydrate and fuel within 30 minutes. Journal post-training session SOP.

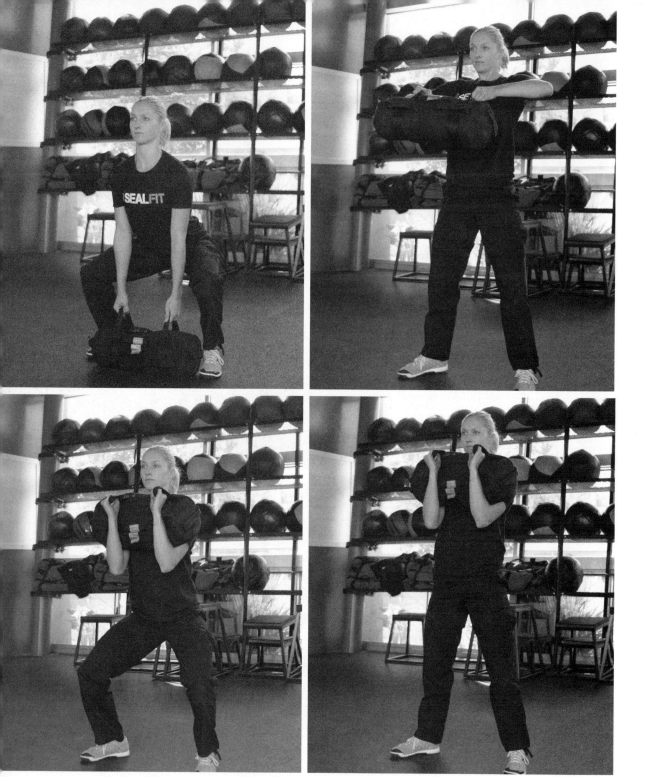

SANDBAG CLEANS

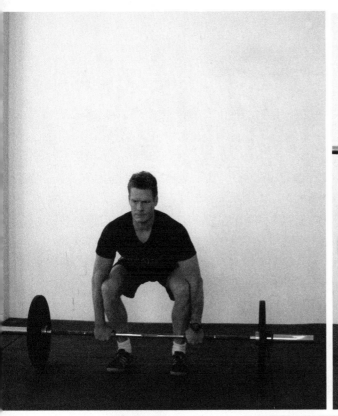
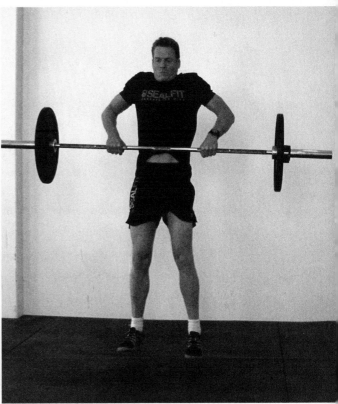
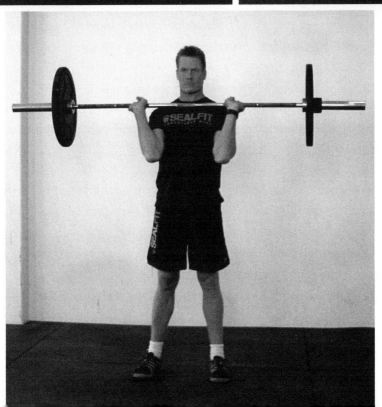

POWER CLEANS

Week 4: Work Capacity

Work capacity cranks the intensity into the red zone. This intense and exhilarating segment takes several months to get used to working as hard as we expect you to in the work capacity sections. SEALFIT defines *work capacity* as "the ability to do more work in less time." An improved work capacity increases power, endurance, speed, and stamina. In other words, you have more horsepower (strength + cardioendurance) and thus have the capacity to perform "more work."

SEALFIT times and conducts work capacity segments like a mini-competition to ensure focus and intensity. You'll quickly develop greater horsepower, confidence, functional fitness, and overall health from combining the training elements of *strength, stamina,* and *work capacity.*

Work capacity "leverages constantly varied functional movements done at high intensity." I credit Coach Greg Glassman, founder of CrossFit, for that powerful combination of words. The real innovation presents these elements as a sport, making the results observable, measurable, and repeatable. Look closer at the three components:

CONSTANT VARIANCE: Variation of exercise types, tools, times, and location. We like to change it up. Routine is the enemy.

FUNCTIONAL MOVEMENTS: Universal motor recruitment pattern movements are found in nature. Avoid artificial movements, such as the dumbbell curl, created in artificial gyms to enhance the artifice of strength for bodybuilding. Bodybuilding training results in "un-training" the body as a system. Keep in mind that a strong muscle is not useful unless it enhances work capacity in the domain of your work, job, or sport. Unless bodybuilding is your actual sport, then hypertrophy training (training for muscle mass) isn't very useful.

HIGH INTENSITY: Timing and treating high-intensity workouts like a sport is brilliant and the ultimate accountability tool. Work capacity is best done with a team or in a coached environment to ensure the quality of movement and the accuracy of count. A word of caution: Timing all workouts can lead to burnout. So I recommend 3 to 4 timed workouts a week, then programming 1 or 2 days off to give your nervous system and cortisol levels a break.

To wrap up SEALFIT On-Ramp Training, we're going to introduce you to a few benchmark workouts, and a TLU (total body, lower body, upper body) strength template. Try your best to perform the work capacities as prescribed, but if you must modify, do so accordingly.

You've already performed your strength movements, so focus on technique and aim to beat your numbers from earlier this month. The first set of 5 strength movements should be light. Increase the weight each set so that the last rep of the last set is near failure (as long as technique is good to go). This week perform 1 total body movement (clean, overhead squat, thruster, etc.), 1 lower-body movement (back squat, front squat, deadlift, etc.), and 1 upper-body movement (press, bench press, weighted pull-up, etc.). This TLU scheme is the strength template used during the On-Ramp program. If you're struggling to keep up with On-Ramp Training, you can continue it through the Online Training at SEALFIT's Web site (www.sealfit.com).

WEEK 4, NEW MOVEMENTS: KB swing, box jump, GHD (glute-hamstring developer) sit-ups.

Teams 'n' Shit

Earn your Trident every day. —SEAL CODE

A HELO sat, rotors spinning up for the air operation training I'd scheduled. A week of fast rope, rappeling, and ocean "rubber duck" jumps lay in store. I really respected our platoon chief, a Vietnam-era SEAL who'd seen more combat and knew more about leadership than I ever would. Now he was nowhere in sight. Later I found him and cornered him awkwardly.

"What's going on, Chief? The guys notice when you miss training. We lead from the front . . . not ask them to do anything we won't do ourselves."

"I know, Cy," he said, looking me straight in the face, completely deadpan. "I was shot down and crash landed in helicopters three times in Nam. Can't stand being exposed to unnecessary air tragedy."

"No shit! I can see your point!" I said, laughing at how he said it. "But this is a new era, with new teammates. I wasn't in Nam with you. Neither were they. You have to prove yourself all over again, each and every day. . . . So do I. You know the deal, Chief. Teams 'n' shit."

The code of SEAL teamwork:

- Loyalty to country, team, and teammate.
- Serve with honor on and off the battlefield.
- Be ready to lead, ready to follow, and never quit.
- Take responsibility for your actions and the actions of your teammates.
- Excel as warriors through discipline and innovation.
- Train for war, fight to win, and defeat our nation's enemies.
- Earn your Trident every day.

"Oh, all right. Darn!" Chief finally said.

The next day he mounted the bird with a smile. The guys noticed. No air tragedy ensued. It cemented their trust.

Chief became one of the most beloved senior enlisted leaders in the teams—always ready with an insane joke or to help a teammate out. He made it a point from then on to always share risk and experience with his teammates.

No matter your level of experience, training with a team accelerates your development. The accountability, planning, shared risk, and shared pain exposes your blind spots. If you don't show up and earn your "trident" every day, you'll remain weak, instead of trading it for strength.

If you've been doing this alone, find someone to do it with you. Journal the change it makes.

BASELINE: pre-SOP and box breathing

- ROM drills
- 3 rounds—200m run, 10x overhead squats (PVC), 10x push-ups
- Shoulder mobility drill

STRENGTH: overhead squat—5 reps × 5 sets

WORK CAPACITY: benchmark—CrossFit's "Nancy"—complete 5 RFT of:

- 400m run
- 15x overhead squats (95#/65#)

DURABILITY: SEALFIT Yoga Short Form B or active stretch. Hydrate and fuel within 30 minutes. Journal post-training session SOP.

TUESDAY [WEEK 4: WORK CAPACITY]

BASELINE: pre-SOP and box breathing

- ROM drills
- 10 minutes of sandbag get-ups (40#/30#)

WORK CAPACITY: complete 15–12–9–6–3 reps:

- KB swings (www.sealfit.com/videos) (16kg/12kg)
- box jumps
- GHD (glute-hamstring developer) sit-ups

DURABILITY: SEALFIT Yoga Short Form A or active stretch. Hydrate and fuel within 30 minutes. Journal post-training session SOP.

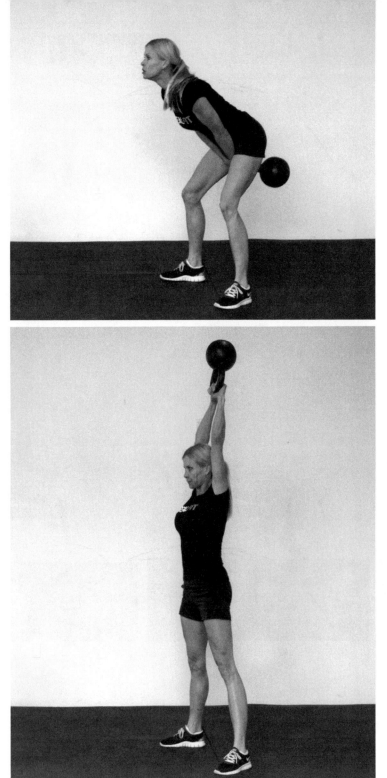

KB SWINGS

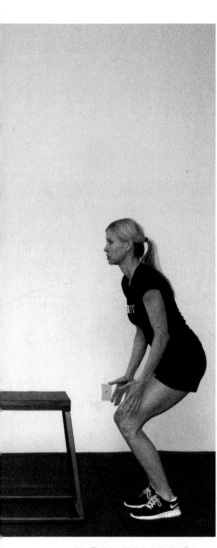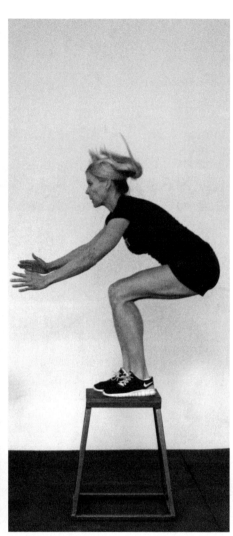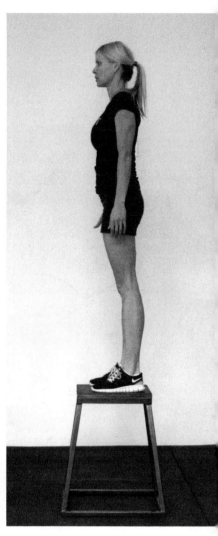

BOX JUMPS

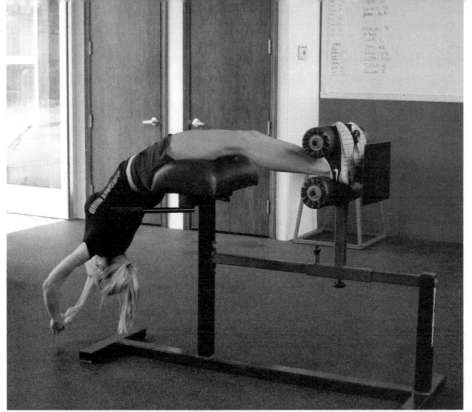

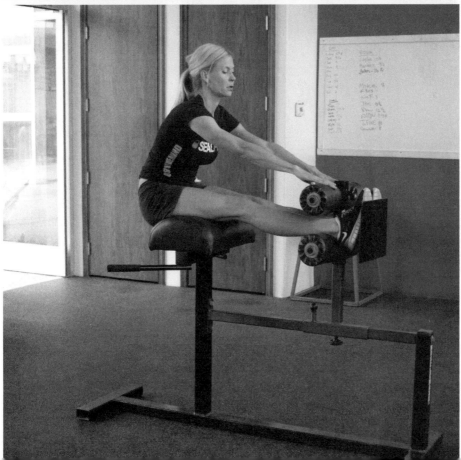

GHD (GLUTE-HAMSTRING DEVELOPER) SIT-UPS

WEDNESDAY [WEEK 4: WORK CAPACITY]

BASELINE: pre-SOP and box breathing

- ROM drills
- 400m run
- 3 rounds—5x air squats, 5x jump squats, 5x push-ups, 5x sit-ups

STRENGTH: back squat—5 reps × 5 sets

WORK CAPACITY: benchmark—CrossFit's "Angie"—for time:

- 100x pull-ups
- 100x push-ups
- 100x sit-ups
- 100x air squats

DURABILITY: SEALFIT Yoga Short Form B or active stretch. Hydrate and fuel within 30 minutes. Journal post-training session SOP.

BASELINE: pre-SOP and box breathing

- ROM drills
- 25 minutes of grinder PT

ENDURANCE: 25 minutes of LSD run, ruck, or swim

DURABILITY: SEALFIT Yoga (any form) or active stretch. Hydrate and fuel within 30 minutes. Journal post-training session SOP.

FRIDAY [WEEK 4: WORK CAPACITY]

BASELINE: pre-SOP and box breathing

- ROM drills
- 250m row
- 15x push presses (45#/35#)
- 250m row
- 15x box jumps (20 inches)

STRENGTH: push press—5 reps × 5 sets

WORK CAPACITY: benchmark—CrossFit's "Fight Gone Bad"—complete 3 rounds:

- 1-minute max wall ball (20#/12#)
- 1-minute max SDHPs (75#/55#)
- 1-minute max box jumps (24 inches or 20 inches)
- 1-minute max push presses (75#/55#)
- 1-minute max calorie row
- 1-minute rest

DURABILITY: SEALFIT Yoga shoulder mobility drill or active stretch. Hydrate and fuel within 30 minutes. Journal post-training session SOP.

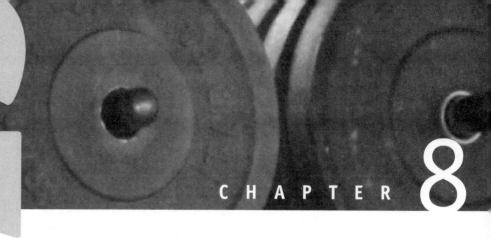

CHAPTER 8

ADVANCED OPERATOR TRAINING

Fortune favors the brave. —PUBLIUS TERENTIUS AFER

W ELCOME TO WHERE THE RUBBER MEETS THE ROAD. THE

8 WEEKS OF THE ADVANCED OPERATOR TRAINING (AOT)

CYCLE IS HOW THIS BOOK GOT ITS NAME. IT'S A HARD-

HITTING, VOLUME-HEAVY TRAINING PROGRAM THAT WILL HELP YOU

TO ACHIEVE AMAZING RESULTS. AS STATED EARLIER, YOU MUST BUILD

THE FOUNDATION BEFORE BARRELING HEADFIRST INTO AOT. IF YOU'RE not ready, stick with the workouts in the Basic Training Program found in Appendix 2 for another month or so.

Strength Cycles in AOT

AOT cycles four primary phases with a de-load week. After the Personal Record (PR) week, you'll reset to the stamina phase and start over. You'll receive a challenge at the end of each month, training all Five Mountains—particularly your kokoro spirit. Not only will they test your mental and spiritual strength, you'll develop tremendous confidence and resolve.

The AOT phases: stamina, strength, power, de-load week, PR.

Each phase is 2 weeks long, progressive, and includes a de-load week in Week 7 prior to your PR week. The de-load week is just that: power down and take a load off your body and mind. Each strength phase is no joke and the de-load week ensures that you recover mentally and physically.

Please be aware that it takes time to condition your body for SEALFIT's volume of work. You'll most likely need occasional additional rest days. I also recommend breaking the sessions in two, several times a week. If you do, perform at least one of the strength days to completion to access its remarkable mental toughness and team-building benefits. As usual, consult your expert within to gauge whether you need a rest day. It's better to rest than grind through a workout with no energy or motivation.

You can stretch the AOT to 11 weeks by adding another de-load week after each phase. You could stretch it further to 16 weeks (or longer) by adding another week to each phase, repeating the last week, but adding an extra set in the (−10 percent) session.

Good luck, and don't hesitate to reach out to us at SEALFIT's Web site (www.sealfit .com) for help. Our online training program could be just the nudge you need. When you've finished, please enroll in the training plans at SEALFIT to continue your training with coaching support.

Week 1: Stamina Phase

Honor

The crowd stood silently as six SEALs hoisted Michael's casket. As they marched toward the line of active duty SEAL teammates, intense pride combined with sadness for their fallen warrior, Michael Monsoor. Unexpected movement disturbed those closest to the line. When the casket reached the first SEAL, he slapped his golden Trident onto the solid mahogany. The next SEAL followed suit.

The wind rustled in the trees. All observed a rare send-off by brothers-in-arms. By the time Michael had traveled the line, over a hundred golden Tridents—a symbol of honor for a SEAL—adorned his casket. Newscasts showed it across the world, a symbol that not many understood, but most appreciated for its beauty.

Michael Monsoor was like you and me—a simple kid who had a dream to be a SEAL. A real team player, he always helped teammates first and worried about his own gear last. He didn't see himself as different—many in the SEAL teams behaved exactly the same way.

In Iraq, Michael volunteered to join an extra mission. It wasn't his turn. He went anyway. An hour later he saw an enemy grenade land a foot away. With no time for them to react, he had a choice: Let it blow and kill his teammates, or take action. His decision was unmistakable. A single word in English fits.

Honor.

Michael jumped on the grenade. His teammates gave him their Tridents and love in return.

Understand the importance of every decision you make from here on, both big and small. Though Michael's sacrifice was above and beyond the call of duty, I'll ask you to jump on a few mental grenades of your own. Those decisions, big and small, will impact your life in ways you may not see initially. Hopefully they won't require the same level of sacrifice as Michael's. But it's important to ask yourself what you *are* willing to sacrifice for the results you're capable of achieving.

It's time to do this thing. Let's represent. *Hooyah!*

MONDAY

BASELINE: pre-SOP and box breathing

- ROM drills
- 400m run
- ROM drills
- work up to 10 RM (repetition maximum) back squat

STRENGTH: back squat—10 reps at −5 percent of 10 RM, 10 reps at −10 percent of 10 RM

STAMINA: chipper, not timed—50x back squats at 50 percent 10 RM, 100x barbell step-ups (15-inch box), 800m buddy carry (If you're without a buddy, walk with a 135# bar on your shoulders for 800m.)

WORK CAPACITY: complete the following for time:

- 30x thrusters (75#/55#)
- 3x rope climbs (15 feet)*
- 20x thrusters (75#/55#)
- 2x rope climbs (15 feet)*
- 10x thrusters (75#/55#)
- 1x rope climb (15 feet)*

DURABILITY: 3-mile run at a moderate pace. 3 rounds—20x weighted sit-ups (45#/25#), 20x back extensions. SEALFIT Yoga Short Form A. Hydrate and fuel within 30 minutes. Journal post-training session SOP.

Note: If you don't have a rope, substitute 6 towel pull-ups for each rope ascent.

TUESDAY [WEEK 1: STAMINA PHASE]

BASELINE: pre-SOP and box breathing

- ROM drills
- 400m run
- ROM drills
- work up to 10 RM push press

STRENGTH: push press—10 reps at −5 percent of 10 RM, 10 reps at −10 percent of 10 RM

STAMINA: 4 rounds, not timed—20x push presses at 50 percent 10 RM, 5x weighted pull-ups AHAP (as heavy as possible), 50m buddy pull with heavy band (If you're without a buddy, substitute 100m sprints with a medicine ball.)

WORK CAPACITY: complete 15 rounds of:

- 1x power snatch + 5x overhead squats*
- 30-second rest

DURABILITY: 15 rounds—30-second max distance row, 30-second rest. 100x 4-count flutter kicks, 100x 4-count wave-offs. SEALFIT Yoga Short Form A. Hydrate and fuel within 30 minutes. Journal post-training session SOP.

Note: Start off light and add weight each round.

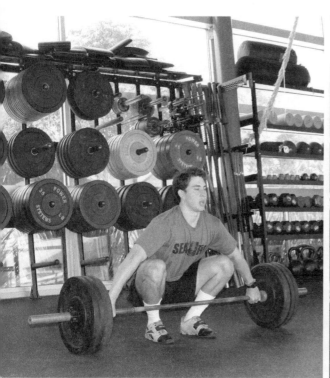

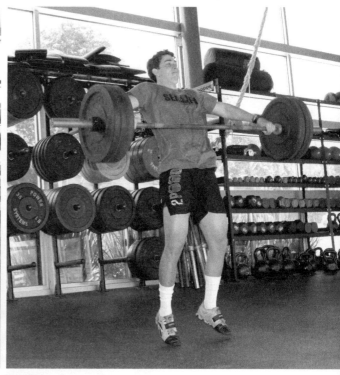

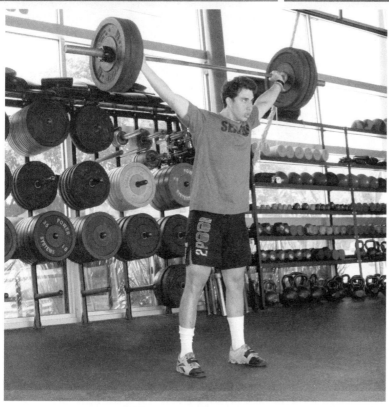

POWER SNATCHES

WEDNESDAY [WEEK 1: STAMINA PHASE]

BASELINE: pre-SOP and box breathing

- ROM drills
- 20 minutes of grinder PT

ENDURANCE: As time allows, LSD run, bike, swim

DURABILITY: SEALFIT Yoga (any form) or active stretch. Hydrate and fuel within 30 minutes. Journal post-training session SOP.

BASELINE: pre-SOP and box breathing

- ROM drills
- 400m run
- work up to 10 RM deadlift

STRENGTH: deadlift—10 reps at −5 percent of 10 RM, 10 reps at −10 percent of 10 RM

STAMINA: chipper, not timed—50x deadlifts at 50 percent 10 RM, 75x SDHP (75#/55#), 400m farmer's carry (55#/35# DBs).

WORK CAPACITY: 50–35–20 reps of:

- wall ball (20#/12#)
- pull-ups
- double-unders

DURABILITY: 2-mile recovery run. 1x max plank hold, 1x max wall sit. SEALFIT Yoga Short Form A. Hydrate and fuel within 30 minutes. Journal post-training session SOP.

FRIDAY [WEEK 1: STAMINA PHASE]

BASELINE: pre-SOP and box breathing

- ROM drills
- 800m run
- work up to 10 RM bench press

STRENGTH: bench press—10 reps at −5 percent of 10 RM, 10 reps at −10 percent of 10 RM

STAMINA: 5 rounds, not timed—15x bench presses at 50 percent 10 RM, 20x alternating arm DB bench presses (35#/25#), 50m overhead weighted walking lunge (45#/25# plate)

WORK CAPACITY: AMRAP in 15 minutes of:

- 10x KB swings (32kg/24kg)
- 10x box jumps (24 or 20 inches)
- 10x ring dips

DURABILITY: 3 rounds—500m row, 400m run, 60-second rest. Then 50x toes to bar. SEALFIT Yoga Short Form B. Hydrate and fuel within 30 minutes. Journal post-training session SOP.

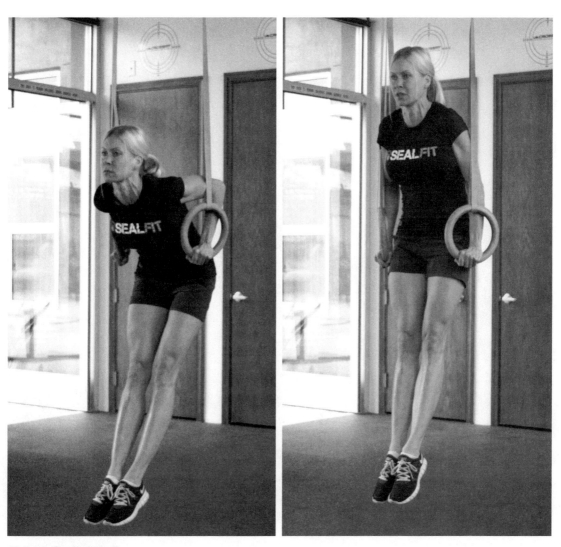

RING DIPS

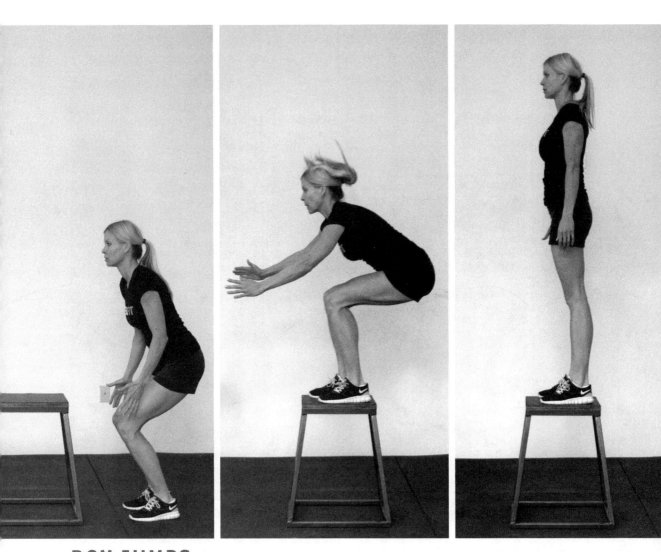

BOX JUMPS

BASELINE: pre-SOP and box breathing

- ROM drill
- 400m run
- 5 rounds of 5x pull-ups, 10x push-ups, 15x air squats

WORK CAPACITY: CrossFit's "Jared"—4 RFT of:

- 800m run
- 40x pull-ups
- 70x push-ups

DURABILITY: 30-minute ruck (use most difficult terrain you have access to). SEALFIT Yoga shoulder mobility drill. Hydrate and fuel within 30 minutes. Journal post-training session SOP.

Week 2: Stamina Phase

Calm Under Pressure

Big Rob swam second to last, near Q. It was dark as hell underneath the hull. I could see my swim buddy but no others. We'd infiltrated the harbor as a single unit, holding a small rope line. I assumed everyone was in position. Anxious to board, I gave the signal to ditch dive rigs and head to the surface, just out of view.

In the darkness, Q got disoriented and failed to plant the magnet on the bottom of the vessel. It plunged to the murky bottom, along with Big Rob and a tangled mess of lines and gear. He had no air supply.

I knew nothing of the unfolding disaster on the surface. We came up one shy in our head count. I asked for a second count, assuming a simple error. Same number. What the heck? How could I lose a guy? The mission was on the verge of being compromised. I quietly called the team together.

"What happened to Big Rob?"

"Not sure, sir," said Q. "I saw him under the ship!"

A sick feeling clawed my stomach. Had I just lost my friend and teammate? I sent swim pairs down into the darkness on breath-hold dives to search the bottom. Nothing.

Tick, tock, tick . . . 4 minutes passed . . .

Suddenly a hand broke the surface, then a head, then the glorious image of Big Rob's face. He was calm, cool, and collected. He smiled.

"Big Rob, checking in, Cy," he said with a nonchalance that defied his near-death experience.

"Thank God. Let's get moving."

In the debrief Big Rob told his side. He was an expert diver and very comfortable in the ocean.

"When the line jerked me to the bottom, I couldn't panic. That'd expend vital energy and oxygen. I conserved it and tried to find a way out."

"How'd you? . . ."

"I started visualizing my body as very calm. My heart slowed down. I scanned my body from head to toe and found the line tangled 'round my web gear. I pulled out my dive knife and sawed myself free. Then I climbed up to the surface, making sure to 'blow and go' to avoid any embolism."

Sixty feet underwater . . . tangled in lines . . . for 4 minutes . . . then a slow climb to oxygen. Just another day as a SEAL. The show must go on.

HOW DO YOU RESPOND IN a crisis? Are you a leader immediately seeking solutions, or do you shrink back, hoping someone else will step up? Do you offer help or demand to be taken care of? The difference between these two opposite attitudes can mean life or death. In more genteel times, it's the difference between living an average and enjoying an extraordinary life.

Strive to maintain a "calm under pressure" mind-set with this week's training plan. Use your breathing to control your mind and body. Visualize yourself as calm and poised, especially during the pain. Make a habit of this attitude. Let it become your character.

MONDAY

BASELINE: pre-SOP and box breathing

- ROM drills
- 500m row, then 2x Frog Complex (75#/45#)*
- work up to 10 RM back squat

STRENGTH: back squat—10 reps at −5 percent of 10 RM, 2 sets × 10 reps at −10 percent of 10 RM

STAMINA: 4 rounds, not timed—20x back squats at 50 percent 10 RM, 25× jump squats, 50m weighted carry (3x 45# plates or 2x 45# plates)

WORK CAPACITY: complete 5 RFT of:

- 5x Frog Complex (115#/75#)*
- 10x burpees

DURABILITY: 4-mile timed run. 100x sit-ups, 100x leg levers. SEALFIT Yoga Short Form A. Hydrate and fuel within 30 minutes. Journal post-training session SOP.

*Note: Frog Complex = squat clean to a thruster + back squat to a thruster in one flowing movement. For the work capacity, 1 Frog Complex is 1 time through the flow (for warm-up, it is 6 cycles for 1 Frog Complex).

BASELINE: pre-SOP and box breathing

- ROM drills
- 500m row
- work up to 10 RM push press

STRENGTH: push press—10 reps at −5 percent of 10 RM, 2 sets × 10 reps at −10 percent of 10 RM

STAMINA: chipper, not timed—50x push presses at 50 percent 10 RM, 75x supine ring rows, 800m buddy carry

WORK CAPACITY: segmented Murph: with 20#/10# vest, for time do:

- 1-mile run
- 10 rounds of 10 pull-ups, 20 push-ups, 30 air squats
- 1-mile run

DURABILITY: SEALFIT Yoga Short Form A. Hydrate and fuel within 30 minutes. Journal post-training session SOP.

WEDNESDAY [WEEK 2: STAMINA PHASE]

BASELINE: pre-SOP and box breathing

- ROM drills
- 20 minutes of grinder PT

ENDURANCE: As time allows, LSD run, bike, swim

DURABILITY: SEALFIT Yoga (any form) or active stretch. Hydrate and fuel within 30 minutes. Journal post-training session SOP.

BASELINE: pre-SOP and box breathing

- ROM drills
- 800M run
- work up to 10 RM deadlift

STRENGTH: deadlift—10 reps at −5 percent of 10 RM, 2 sets × 10 reps at −10 percent of 10 RM

STAMINA: 5 rounds, not timed—15x deadlifts at 50 percent 10 RM, 20x box jumps (24 or 20 inches), 50m bear crawl

WORK CAPACITY: complete the following for time:

- 15x thrusters (135#/95#)
- 200m run
- 20x thrusters (95#/65#)
- 400m run
- 30x thrusters (65#/45#)
- 800m run

DURABILITY: 5k-meter row. 100x GHD sit-ups. SEALFIT Yoga Short Form A. Hydrate and fuel within 30 minutes. Journal post-training session SOP.

FRIDAY [WEEK 2: STAMINA PHASE]

BASELINE: pre-SOP and box breathing

- ROM drills
- 500m row
- work up to 10 RM bench press

STRENGTH: bench press—10 reps at −5 percent of 10 RM, 2 sets × 10 reps at −10 percent of 10 RM

STAMINA: chipper, not timed—50x bench presses at 50 percent 10 RM, 75x plyometric push-ups,* 400m walking lunge

WORK CAPACITY: AMRAP 20 minutes of:

- 250m row
- 15x DB squat cleans (2x 40#/25# DB)

DURABILITY: 1x 800m sprint, 1x 400m sprint, 1x 200m sprint, 1x 100m sprint (1:1 work to rest). SEALFIT Yoga Short Form A. Hydrate and fuel within 30 minutes. Journal post-training session SOP.

*Note: Plyometric push-ups—the entire body comes off the ground on each rep.

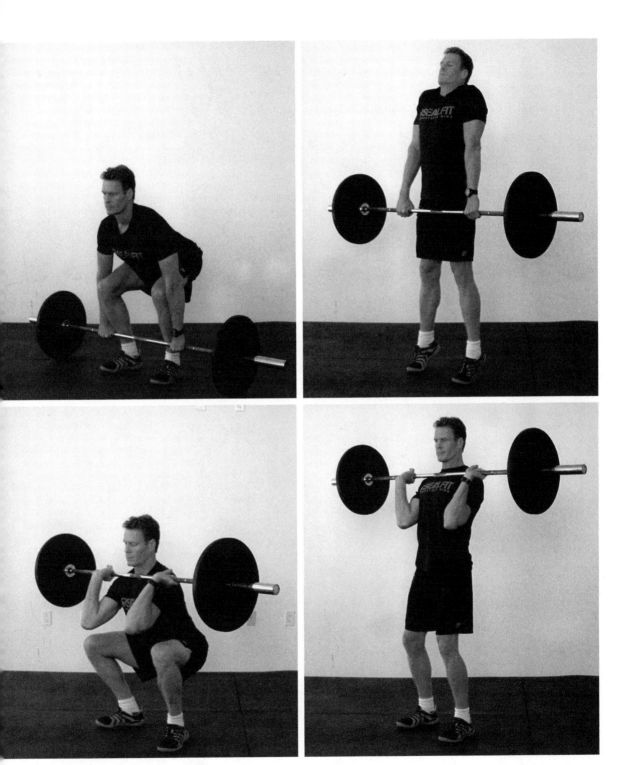

SQUAT CLEANS

SATURDAY [WEEK 2: STAMINA PHASE]

BASELINE: pre-SOP and box breathing

- ROM drills
- 10 minutes of sandbag get-ups

WORK CAPACITY: complete the following as fast as possible:

- 800m run
- 10 rounds—10x KB swings (24kg/16kg), 10x push-ups, 10x sit-ups, 10x air squats
- 800m run

DURABILITY: 30-minute trail or beach run. 100x 4-count flutter kicks, 100x leg levers. SEALFIT Yoga Short Form A. Hydrate and fuel within 30 minutes. Journal post-training session SOP.

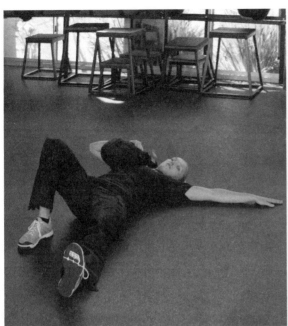
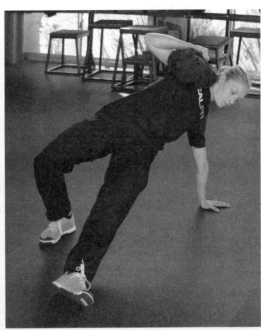
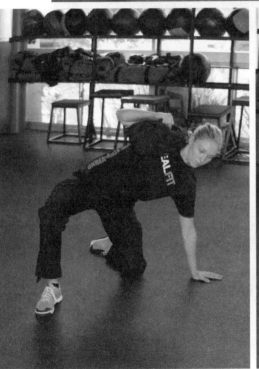
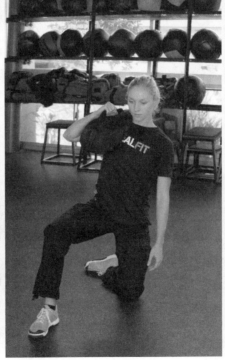
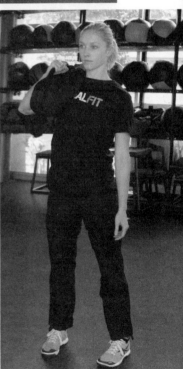

SANDBAG GET-UPS

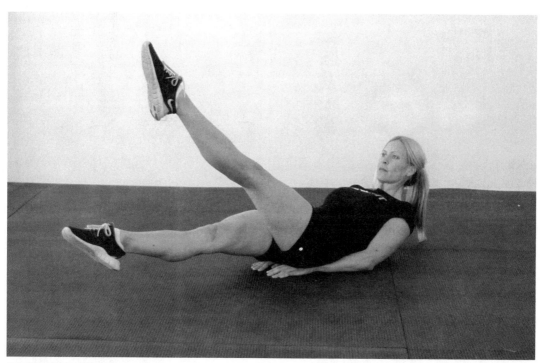

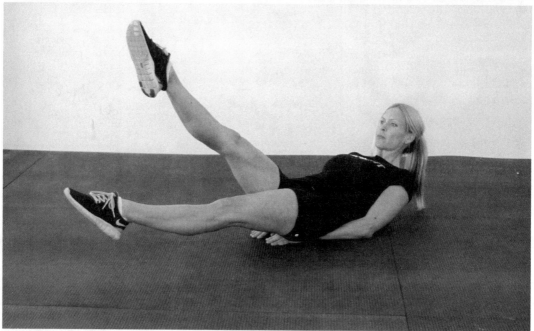

FLUTTER KICKS

Week 3: Strength Phase

More About Strength Training

Not a day goes by that a Navy SEAL isn't required to lift and carry a heavy load over a distance. If you focus to exclusion on a single-mode, monostructural sport such as running, biking, or triathlon training, you'll have trouble handling heavy loads and could be a liability to your team.

Strength training isn't complicated or sexy. It's hard work. But when properly executed, it's fun, rewarding, and provides great team-training opportunities. Body-weight exercises are certainly valuable, but they're limited in their ability to develop significant strength gains. If you lack the necessary equipment for SEALFIT's prescribed strength training, you can complete most of the work with a sandbag or makeshift equipment.

Grit

Chief Smith knew this wouldn't turn out well. The two "nonteam" guys insisted they carry all the crap they'd brought for the op.

"Frank," Smith said to one of the agents, "why don't you leave half that shit here? You're not going to be able to get all that gear up the hill, and you don't need it anyhow."

"I got it, man. Don't worry 'bout us."

By the time Smith and the team passed through the ravine and reached the foot of the mountain, the sun had set. They gazed up at the snow-covered landscape and the moon cresting over the ridgeline in the distance. They started up, breaking brush along the way. Smith set a blistering pace that was normal for him and his teammates. The augmentees started to fall behind.

After a couple of hours, the chief stopped to take a break and check in with his team. When the other guys caught up, he went to Frank.

"How you guys doing?"

"This is . . . uh . . . hard terrain, I had no . . . uh . . . idea."

No shit, Sherlock, this is Afghanistan. Smith didn't say it, but his eyes did.

"I don't think I can haul this gear anymore," Frank gasped.

His teammate agreed. Chief Smith turned and started walking up the hill. He wasn't going to let these guys hold them back from their objective. They arrived at their rendezvous point in 4 hours. The augmentees chugged up a half hour later, minus their gear.

With just a look, Chief Smith and his SEAL teammate headed back down the hill. Finding the ditched gear, they put it on their backs and hauled it up. They set the gear down near the sleeping guys, without saying a word.

GRIT IS THE ONLY WORD in English that comes close to describing the mind-set of Chief Smith and his teammates. It evokes images of gnarly cowboys or ranch hands working in extreme conditions. It means to thrive in adversity, to revel in the learning that accompanies doing very hard things. The cool thing about grit is that it develops like a callus. The more you lean into the hard things, the grittier your character becomes. If you slack off, you lose it. Grit is earned.

Earn it. Hit each training session like your hair's on fire. Bring that same attitude to everything you do. If you don't possess passion for your training, fake it 'til you make it. Find your limits and shatter them. You don't want someone else with more grit to carry your load.

BASELINE: pre-SOP and box breathing

- ROM drills
- 800m run
- work up to 5 RM back squat

STRENGTH: back squat—5 reps at −5 percent of 5 RM, 2 sets × 5 reps at −10 percent of 5 RM

STAMINA: 5 rounds, not timed—15x back squats at 45 percent 5 RM, 25x 4-count mountain climbers, max time hanging towel hold (Put a towel over a pull-up bar, and see how long you can hang before your grip fails.)

WORK CAPACITY: complete 3 RFT of:

- 21x thrusters (95#/65#)
- 15x KB swings (32kg/24kg)
- 12x pull-ups
- 9x burpees

DURABILITY: 3 rounds for max distance—60-second row, 60-second active rowing rest, 45-second row, 45-second active rowing rest, 30-second row, 30-second active rowing rest. 100x 4-count flutter kicks, 100x leg levers. SEALFIT Yoga Short Form B. Hydrate and fuel within 30 minutes. Journal post-training session SOP.

WEEK 3: STRENGTH PHASE

TUESDAY [WEEK 3: STRENGTH PHASE]

BASELINE: pre-SOP and box breathing

- ROM drills
- 500m run
- work up to 5 RM push press

STRENGTH: push press—5 reps at −5 percent of 5 RM, 2 sets × 5 reps at −10 percent of 5 RM

STAMINA: chipper, not timed—50x push presses at 45 percent 5 RM, 100x jumping pull-ups, 800m farmer's walk (135#/95# up to body weight)*

WORK CAPACITY: 1 round—3 minutes max effort at each station, 1-minute rest between each station:

- max calorie row
- overhead squat (95#/65#)
- ball slam
- sit-up
- 800m run as fast as possible

DURABILITY: 2-mile recovery run. 3 rounds—10x strict toes to bars, 10x weighted back extensions (45#/25#). SEALFIT Yoga Short Form A. Hydrate and fuel within 30 minutes. Journal post-training session SOP.

*Note: Farmer's walk = put a barbell on your back in the back squat rack position and walk 800m.

BASELINE: pre-SOP and box breathing

- ROM drills
- 20 minutes of grinder PT

ENDURANCE: As time allows, LSD run, bike, swim

DURABILITY: SEALFIT Yoga (any form) or active stretch. Hydrate and fuel within 30 minutes. Journal post-training session SOP.

THURSDAY [WEEK 3: STRENGTH PHASE]

BASELINE: pre-SOP and box breathing

- ROM drills
- 800m run
- work up to 5 RM deadlift

STRENGTH: deadlift—5 reps at −5 percent of 5 RM, 2 sets × 5 reps at −10 percent of 5 RM

STAMINA: 4 rounds, not timed—20x deadlifts at 45 percent 5 RM, 10x one-legged box jumps each leg (15 inches), max time chin above the bar hold (Do a pull-up and see how long you can hold your chin above the bar.)

WORK CAPACITY: 5 rounds for completion:

- max handstand push-ups (www.sealfit.com/videos)*
- 400m run*

DURABILITY: 10x 50m sprint (starting position = lying down with stomach on the deck). 100x sit-ups, 100x wave-offs. SEALFIT Yoga shoulder mobility drill. Hydrate and fuel within 30 minutes. Journal post-training session SOP.

Note: Rest as needed between rounds.

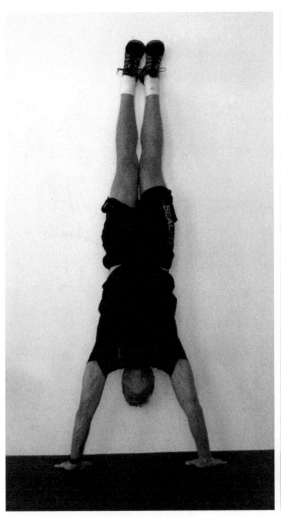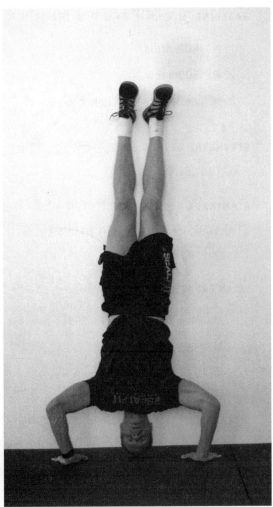

HANDSTAND PUSH-UPS

FRIDAY [WEEK 3: STRENGTH PHASE]

BASELINE: pre-SOP and box breathing

- ROM drills
- 500m row
- work up to 5 RM bench press

STRENGTH: bench press—5 reps at −5 percent of 5 RM, 2 sets × 5 reps at −10 percent of 5 RM

STAMINA: chipper, not timed—50x bench presses at 45 percent 5 RM, 100x close-grip bench press (45#/30#), 400m weighted walking lunge (55#/35#)

WORK CAPACITY: 10–9–8–7–6–5–4–3–2–1 reps of:

- Man Makers (2x 35#/25#) (www.sealfit.com/videos)
- pull-ups
- 2x sit-ups

DURABILITY: 3-mile run at a moderate pace. 1x max plank hold, 1x max wall sit. SEALFIT Yoga Short Form A. Hydrate and fuel within 30 minutes. Journal post-training session SOP.

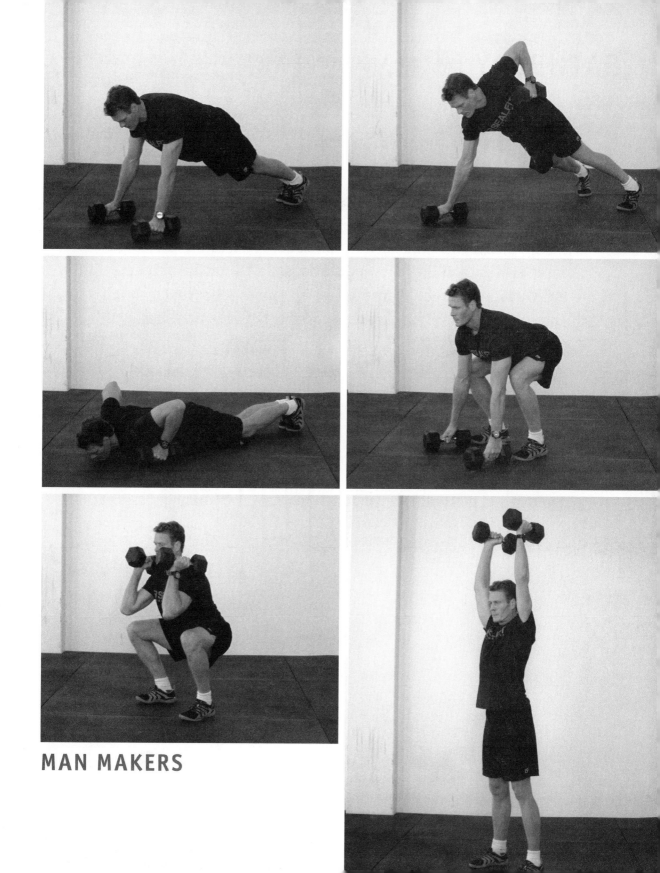

MAN MAKERS

SATURDAY [WEEK 3: STRENGTH PHASE]

BASELINE: pre-SOP and box breathing

- ROM drills
- 2 rounds of 400m run and 15x sandbag get-ups

WORK CAPACITY: CrossFit's "Tabata Gone Bad." Complete a full Tabata interval at each of the following stations. Rest 1 minute between each Tabata interval. Tabata interval = 8 rounds, 20 seconds work, 10 seconds rest. Transition as fast as possible between exercises.

- double unders
- row
- push press (75#/55#)
- jumping lunges

DURABILITY: 30-minute trail or beach run. SEALFIT Yoga Short Form A. Hydrate and fuel within 30 minutes. Journal post-training session SOP.

Week 4: Strength Phase

Drive

I met Jeff Kraus at SEAL Team 3, where we boxed once a week for fun.

"Jeff, how'd you end up a SEAL anyhow?" I asked during a sparring session.

"Well, I got out of the Army and went to college. But I got bored quickly in the regular workforce. So I decided to join the Navy."

"What'd you do in the Army?"

"I was a Ranger . . . then a Green Beret."

Holy cow—the trifecta of Special Operations Forces! I'd known some SEALs who got sent to Ranger School or the Special Forces "Q" Course (the Green Beret's course). But never had I heard of someone actually serving as a Ranger, a Green Beret, *and* a SEAL.

"Boy, Jeff, you must be driven!"

He smiled. Then he socked me upside the head with his gloved hand to restart the bout.

IT'S EASY TO GET MOTIVATED about something, only to forget it when the next shiny thing comes along. Being driven is something else. It doesn't need a parade. You can't drum it up with a Red Bull.

Passion for excellence and a sense of purpose drove Jeff to be more than just any military operator. He simply wouldn't stand for anything less. Day after day he saw the result of missions accomplished and new skills developed. It fueled a deeper belief in his abilities, a humble expectation of the need for him to be exceptional.

Want to become more like Jeff? So do I. Build your confidence and certainty. Start by getting driven to accomplish modest goals that you're passionate about. Then commit that passion to a purpose that's bigger than you. What purpose will you choose to fuel your passion?

CrossFit Games stars Lindsey Valenzuela and Kristan Clever had the gumption to attend Kokoro Camp to better themselves. Their drive shows in their passion for their fledgling sport. Day after day they see themselves as inspirations for others, serving as role models for you and me.

Check into your passion and purpose daily. When you act in alignment with both, you'll find a drive like Jeff's, like Lindsey's, like Kristan's. Develop some drive in this week's training. Hit it hard and have some fun!

BASELINE: pre-SOP and box breathing

- ROM drills
- 800m run
- work up to 5 RM back squat

STRENGTH: back squat—5 reps at −5 percent of 5 RM, 3 sets × 5 reps at −10 percent of 5 RM

STAMINA: chipper, not timed—50x back squats at 45 percent 5 RM, 100x Bulgarian split squat (a lunge with the back foot on a box), 800m buddy carry

WORK CAPACITY: complete 40–30–20–10 reps of:

- DB thrusters (35#/25#)
- knees to elbows

DURABILITY: 4-mile timed run. SEALFIT Yoga Short Form A. Hydrate and fuel within 30 minutes. Journal post-training session SOP.

TUESDAY [WEEK 4: STRENGTH PHASE]

BASELINE: pre-SOP and box breathing

- ROM drills
- 400m run
- work up to 5 RM push press

STRENGTH: push press—5 reps at −5 percent of 5 RM, 3 sets × 5 reps at −10 percent of 5 RM

STAMINA: 5 rounds, not timed—15x push presses at 45 percent 5 RM, 20x alternating arm KB floor presses (35#/26#), 50m buddy pull with heavy band

WORK CAPACITY: wearing weighted vest, perform 3 RFT of:

- 500m row
- 21x box jumps (24 or 20 inches)
- 12x pull-ups

DURABILITY: 2x 800m sprint (1:1 work to rest), 100x leg levers, 100x wave-offs. SEALFIT Yoga Short Form B. Hydrate and fuel within 30 minutes. Journal post-training session SOP.

BASELINE: pre-SOP and box breathing

- ROM drills
- 20 minutes of grinder PT

ENDURANCE: As time allows, LSD run, bike, swim

DURABILITY: SEALFIT Yoga (any form) or active stretch. Hydrate and fuel within 30 minutes. Journal post-training session SOP.

THURSDAY [WEEK 4: STRENGTH PHASE]

BASELINE: pre-SOP and box breathing

- ROM drills
- 500m row
- work up to 5 RM deadlift

STRENGTH: deadlift—5 reps at −5 percent of 5 RM, 3 sets × 5 reps at −10 percent of 5 RM

STAMINA: chipper, not timed—50x deadlift at 45 percent 5 RM, 75x KB SDHPs (24kg/16kg), 400m farmer's carry (55#/35#)

WORK CAPACITY: complete the following for time:

- 1-mile run
- 30x clean and jerks (135#/95#)
- 1-mile run

DURABILITY: 2,000m row. SEALFIT Yoga shoulder mobility drill. Hydrate and fuel within 30 minutes. Journal post-training session SOP.

BASELINE: pre-SOP and box breathing

- ROM drills
- 800m run
- work up to 5 RM bench press

STRENGTH: bench press—5 reps at −5 percent of 5 RM, 3 sets × 5 reps at −10 percent of 5 RM

STAMINA: 4 rounds, not timed—20x bench presses at 45 percent 5 RM, 75x supine ring rows, 25m weighted overhead walking lunge (45#/25#)

WORK CAPACITY: AMRAP in 15 minutes of:

- 5x squat snatches (95#/65#)
- 30x wall balls (20#/12#)

DURABILITY: 6x 200m sprints (60-second interval). 100x 4-count flutter kicks, 100x leg levers. SEALFIT Yoga Short Form A. Hydrate and fuel within 30 minutes. Journal post-training session SOP.

SATURDAY [WEEK 4: STRENGTH PHASE]

BASELINE: pre-SOP and box breathing

- ROM drills
- 3 rounds—200m run, 10x wall balls, 10x jumping pull-ups, 10x sit-ups

WORK CAPACITY: complete the following for time:

- 2-mile run
- 10 rounds—5x pull-ups, 10x push-ups, 15x air squats
- 2-mile run

DURABILITY: 30-minute weight vest or light ruck run. SEALFIT Yoga Short Form A. Hydrate and fuel within 30 minutes. Journal post-training session SOP.

Challenges

Start by doing what's necessary, then what's possible, and suddenly you are doing the impossible. —ST. FRANCIS OF ASSISI

Congratulations on completing your first month of Advanced Operator Training! It's time for your first challenge. It will train your kokoro, find your 20x, and function as a terrific teambuilding event. "Do today what others won't, do tomorrow what others can't." Don't just know this as a great quote, seek to live it. Use it as a benchmark to map your future progress. The workout called Murph—named after Michael Murphy, a fallen Navy SEAL—is a challenging benchmark workout.

Choose one of the listed benchmark challenges below. Next month you will have a different list. If you're stretching your phases out, you'll need to choose more challenges to complete one every calendar month. Substitute any for a workout. My team likes to perform benchmark workouts and challenges on Saturdays, but you can do them whenever they work for your schedule. It's a good idea to take it easy the day after. Of course, consult your physician prior, *blah, blah, blah,* and don't do anything beyond your capabilities. As if you knew what those were . . .

FOR TIME
(DO 1 OF THESE, NOT ALL OF THEM—EVEN I AM NOT THAT CRAZY!):

- 1,000 push-ups
- 1,000 sit-ups
- 1,000 pull-ups
- 100 rope ascents
- 1,000 8-count body builders
- 1,000 burpees
- 100 Curtis Ps or 100 Man Makers
- 1-mile walking lunge wearing a 20# weight vest

These challenges may seem insurmountable if you're new to physical training, but rest assured, they're achievable and rewarding when completed. If you follow the principles of

SEALFIT and don't have any physical limitations outside of the norm, you can do this! Don't hesitate to scale the challenges. The older you get, the more you may need to scale down or establish realistic time expectations, but that doesn't mean they shouldn't be done. When you're ready, execute the first one. Complete it 1 rep, 1 step, 1 breath at a time. You'll shatter your paradigm and build extreme confidence in your ability to push through self-imposed limitations. You'll possess another useful training tool in your growing toolbox.

Now get to it. Your 20x factor awaits!

Week 5: Power Phase

Fire in the Belly

In certain rare people a fire burns brightly in their belly. This fire stokes their courage and passion in a way that allows them to persevere in the most adverse conditions—when all cards are stacked against them. This is not to be confused with confidence. No, a fire in the belly is not born of unique skill or great physical strength; rather, it comes from a deep willpower tinged with humility. This fire in the belly allows them to not just survive, but to thrive with any challenge.

I read these words and then presented the Fire in the Belly award to the only female participant in Kokoro Camp 27. With shock and a tear in her eye, Ally stepped forward while her teammates cheered. They weren't surprised in the least, having witnessed the same thing as my coaching staff and I had.

BECOMING A PHYSICAL STUD IS easy. Unless you have a serious, preexisting limitation, quality time at the gym and on-the-field training eventually develops studliness. Though it makes you more durable, it doesn't make you a leader and won't guarantee your survival in a major crisis.

Ally's fitness didn't set her apart. She possessed mental toughness, but so did the other trainees. What separated Ally was the fire in her belly that nothing could smother. She soldiered on under the most adverse conditions. I observed these character traits:

- While others winced, she embraced the suck and turned pain into performance with a smile.
- While others turned within, she focused on her teammates, giving them encouragement and support.

- While others leapt with fear from the unknown, she jumped forward with the faith that things would be okay.

- While others expected to do well, she expected nothing. Her mind, body, and spirit readied to fight every inch.

Fire in the belly. Could that be the same as kokoro spirit—that obscure goal of ours to merge hearts and minds in action? It just might be. Without knowing it, Ally came with a kokoro spirit forged and ready to spring into action. The experience merely validated her preparation and character. She stepped up to an entirely new level of performance—one fueled by her spirit and not her body.

What can you do to cultivate your fire in the belly? Find deep meaning in serving. Out of love and respect take your eyes off yourself and place them on your teammates. This eradicates self-centered and cowardly behavior, replacing it with humility and courage.

Hooyah! Fire in the belly!

BASELINE: pre-SOP and box breathing

- ROM drills
- 800m run
- work up to 3 RM back squat

STRENGTH: back squat—3 reps at −5 percent of 3 RM, 3 sets × 3 reps at −10 percent of 3 RM

STAMINA: chipper, not timed—50x back squats at 40 percent 3 RM, 75x barbell jump squats, 800m overhead carry (45#/25#)

WORK CAPACITY: complete the following for time:

- 30x burpee box jumps (24 or 20 inches)
- 30x toes to bars
- 30x push jerks (135#/95#)
- 1,000m row

DURABILITY: 4-mile timed run (goal is under 32 minutes). 5 rounds—60-second plank, 60-second back extensions. SEALFIT Yoga Short Form B. Hydrate and fuel within 30 minutes. Journal post-training session SOP.

TUESDAY [WEEK 5: POWER PHASE]

BASELINE: pre-SOP and box breathing

- ROM drills
- 500m row
- work up to 3 RM push press

STRENGTH: push press—3 reps at −5 percent of 3 RM, 3 sets × 3 reps at −10 percent of 3 RM

STAMINA: 5 rounds, not timed—15x push presses at 40 percent 3 RM, 20x dips, 25m overhead weighted lunge (45#/25#)

WORK CAPACITY: CrossFit's "Amanda." Complete 9–7–5 reps of:

- muscle-ups (www.sealfit.com/videos)*
- snatch (135#/95#)

DURABILITY: 8x 250m row (60-second interval). 100x sit-ups, 100x leg levers. SEALFIT Yoga shoulder mobility drill. Hydrate and fuel within 30 minutes. Journal post-training session SOP.

Note: Substitute 6x pull-ups and 6x dips for each muscle-up if you can't perform the muscle-up.

MUSCLE-UPS

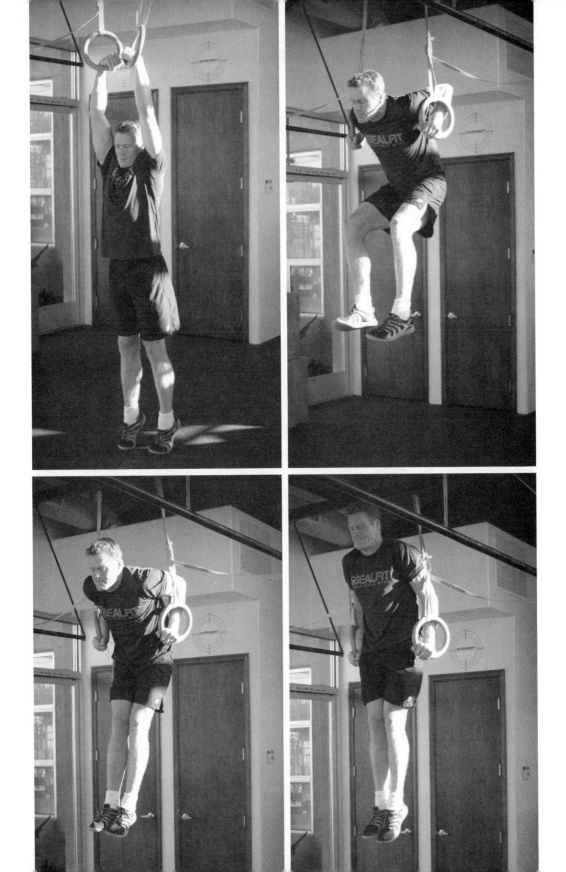

WEDNESDAY [WEEK 5: POWER PHASE]

BASELINE: pre-SOP and box breathing

- ROM drills
- 20 minutes of grinder PT

ENDURANCE: As time allows, LSD run, bike, swim

DURABILITY: SEALFIT Yoga (any form) or active stretch. Hydrate and fuel within 30 minutes. Journal post-training session SOP.

BASELINE: pre-SOP and box breathing

- ROM drills
- 800m run
- work up to 3 RM deadlift

STRENGTH: deadlift—3 reps at −5 percent of 3 RM, 3 sets × 3 reps at −10 percent of 3 RM

STAMINA: chipper, not timed—50x deadlifts at 40 percent 3 RM, 75x barbell SDHPs (75#/55#), 800m buddy carry

WORK CAPACITY: complete 4 rounds for:

- 400m run
- 15x power cleans (115#/75#)
- 15x ring dips

DURABILITY: 2-mile recovery run. 3 rounds—10x 1-arm weighted sit-ups (35#/26#), 20x Russian twist (25#/15#). SEALFIT Yoga Short Form A. Hydrate and fuel within 30 minutes. Journal post-training session SOP.

FRIDAY [WEEK 5: POWER PHASE]

BASELINE: pre-SOP and box breathing

- ROM drills
- 500m row
- work up to 3 RM bench press

STRENGTH: bench press—3 reps at −5 percent of 3 RM, 3 sets × 3 reps at −10 percent of 3 RM

STAMINA: 4 rounds, not timed—20x bench presses at 40 percent 3 RM, 10x 1-arm DB bent-over row (each arm), 60-second farmer's carry (55#/35#)

WORK CAPACITY: complete the following for time:

- 100x wall balls (20#/12#)
- 75x KB swings (24kg/16kg)
- 50x jumping lunges
- 25x pull-ups

DURABILITY: 1-mile sprint. 50x evil wheels (you can also use a barbell for these). SEALFIT Yoga hip mobility drill. Hydrate and fuel within 30 minutes. Journal post-training session SOP.

BASELINE: pre-SOP and box breathing

- ROM drills
- 30–20–10 reps of air squats, push-ups, sit-ups

WORK CAPACITY: in a team of two, complete as fast as possible. Only one person can be working at a time. Partner is in the lean and rest position while the other is working.*

- 800m run together
- 100x ball slams (30#/20#)
- 800m run together
- 100x sledge strikes (Substitute KB snatches (35#/30#) for the sledge strikes if you lack the equipment.)

DURABILITY: 30-minute ruck. SEALFIT Yoga Short Form A. Hydrate and fuel within 30 minutes. Journal post-training session SOP.

*Note: If you lack a partner, perform the work prescribed solo and enjoy the bonus.

Week 6: Power Phase

Feed the Courage Dog

What dog are you feeding, Mark?

I was in the middle of a CrossFit Games workout in the Master's division Open Tournament when I asked myself this question. The 135-pound snatch was crushing me after all the burpees. I kicked the bar after my third failed attempt. The fear dog growled as the clock ticked down to the 17-minute deadline . . .

TWO HUNGRY DOGS VIE FOR your attention every moment. The fear dog growls and gets fed a lot, especially when things aren't going well. The courage dog humbly waits for attention and often goes hungry. Which dog are you feeding? Listen to your answer. It illuminates deep patterns of a positive or negative bias toward life. You can train yourself to have a positive bias at all times. It will make a big difference. Here's how.

Slow things down enough to pay attention to what's going on inside your noggin. Inhale three deep breaths when you feel uncertain, agitated, or fearful. As you breathe, ask the question "What dog am I feeding?" Notice how you feel right then. Reflect on which thoughts dominated your mind moments before. If you feel anxiety, fear, or negativity, your internal dialogue and imagery was negative. Interrupt it immediately and redirect the energy to something positive. Develop a *power statement* you can use like:

- Easy day!
- I got this!
- Feeling good!

These statements replace negative thought patterns with a powerful and positively charged one. Then maintain that mood with these three techniques:

- **POSTURE:** If you feed the courage dog, you stand up straight, hold your head high, breathe deeply, and charge your body with energy. If the fear dog predominates, you shrink with your head down, shirk direct eye contact, and avoid taking responsibility. Your body's posture takes your mind higher into hope or even deeper into despair.

- **VISUALIZING:** You stimulate your muscles at a subtle physiological level when you see yourself as powerful or weak in your mind's eye. The fear dog projects images of weakness and failure. The courage dog offers images of power and success. Charge them with emotion, and your body will embrace the mind's reality!

- **MANTRA:** The word has some baggage, I agree, but it's still useful. It's simply a positive affirmation, like a software program you run in your mind's background. My two main mantras are: "Day by day, in every way, I am getting better and better" and "Feeling good, looking good, ought to be in Hollywood." They mean a lot to me and keep the fear dog from barking.

Meanwhile back at my CrossFit Games challenge . . .

I PAUSED, TOOK THREE DEEP breaths, and stared at nothing in particular. I pictured myself getting the next snatch above my head, and thought, *I've got this. Easy day. Feeling good. Throw your heart into it, Mark . . . Let's go!*

The fear of failing slipped away. I approached the bar with new determination. I would do the best I possibly could. Fear would not dominate me. The snatch attempt was good. Back on track.

WHAT DOG ARE YOU FEEDING now? Throw that courage dog a juicy steak. Move with positivity in your training and beyond.

MONDAY

BASELINE: pre-SOP and box breathing

- ROM drills
- 500m row
- work up to 3 RM back squat

STRENGTH: back squat—3 reps at —5 percent of 3 RM, 4 sets × 3 reps at —10 percent of 3 RM

STAMINA: 5 rounds, not timed—15x back squats at 40 percent 3 RM, 20x 1-legged box jump (15 inch), 25m crab walk

WORK CAPACITY: 4 rounds AMRAP in 3 minutes of:*

- 3x thrusters (95#/65#)
- 6x KB swings (55#/35#)
- 9x toes to bars
- 1-minute rest between each round

DURABILITY: 2x 800m sprint (rest 2 minutes between sprints). 100x 4-count flutter kicks, 100x leg levers. SEALFIT Yoga Short Form B. Hydrate and fuel within 30 minutes. Journal post-training session SOP.

*Note: Do as many rounds of 3x thrusters, 6x KB swings, and 9x toes to bars in 3 minutes as possible. Take a 1-minute rest, then repeat 3 more times.

BASELINE: pre-SOP and box breathing

- ROM drills
- 800m run
- work up to 3 RM push press

STRENGTH: push press—3 reps at −5 percent of 3 RM, 4 sets × 3 reps at −10 percent of 3 RM

STAMINA: chipper, not timed—50x push presses at 40 percent 3 RM, 75x supine ring pull-ups, 400m sandbag walking lunge (sandbag held in front rack position—like you are carrying a log)

WORK CAPACITY: complete the following for time:

- 1,000m row
- 12x power snatches (95#/65#)
- 750m row
- 9x power snatches (95#/65#)
- 500m row
- 6x power snatches (95#/65#)
- 250m row
- 3x power snatches (95#/65#)

DURABILITY: 3 rounds—15x weighted sit-ups (45#/25#), 45-second side bridge (perform 45 seconds on each side). SEALFIT Yoga Short Form B. Hydrate and fuel within 30 minutes. Journal post-training session SOP.

WEDNESDAY [WEEK 6: POWER PHASE]

BASELINE: pre-SOP and box breathing

- ROM drills
- 20 minutes of grinder PT

ENDURANCE: As time allows, LSD run, bike, swim

DURABILITY: SEALFIT Yoga or active stretch. Hydrate and fuel within 30 minutes. Journal post-training session SOP.

BASELINE: pre-SOP and box breathing

- ROM drills
- 500m row
- work up to 3 RM deadlift

STRENGTH: deadlift—3 reps at −5 percent of 3 RM, 4 sets × 3 reps at −10 percent of 3 RM

STAMINA: 4 rounds, not timed—20x deadlifts at 40 percent 3 RM, 30x jumping lunges, max time towel hold (Drape a towel over a pull-up bar and hang on as long as you can.)

WORK CAPACITY: complete the following for time:

- 400m run
- 3 rounds—5x clean and jerks (135#/95#), 10x chest-to-bar pull-ups, 15x burpees
- 400m run

DURABILITY: 3-mile run at a moderate pace. 100x wave-offs. SEALFIT Yoga Short Form A. Hydrate and fuel within 30 minutes. Journal post-training session SOP.

FRIDAY [WEEK 6: POWER PHASE]

BASELINE: pre-SOP and box breathing

- ROM drills
- 800m run
- work up to 3 RM bench press

STRENGTH: bench press—3 reps at −5 percent of 3 RM, 4 sets × 3 reps at −10 percent of 3 RM

STAMINA: chipper, not timed—50x bench presses at 40 percent 3 RM, 60x renegade row (25#/15#), 800m buddy carry

WORK CAPACITY: complete 21–15–9 reps of:

- front squats (155#/115#)
- sandbag get-ups

DURABILITY: 8x hill sprints. (If you don't have access to a hill, substitute stair sprints or 200m sprints at a 30-second interval.) 1x max plank hold. SEALFIT Yoga hip mobility drill. Hydrate and fuel within 30 minutes. Journal post-training session SOP.

BASELINE: pre-SOP and box breathing

- ROM drills
- 2 rounds—400m run, 15x KB swings (16kg/12kg)

WORK CAPACITY: CrossFit's "Filthy Fifty"—for time do:

- 50x box jumps (24 inches/20 inches)
- 50x jumping pull-ups
- 50x KB swings (16kg/12kg)
- 50x walking lunge steps
- 50x knees to elbows
- 50x push presses (45#/35#)
- 50x back extensions
- 50x wall ball shots (20#/12#)
- 50x burpees
- 50x double unders

DURABILITY: 30-minute trail or beach run. Max sit-ups in 2 minutes, max push-ups in 2 minutes. SEALFIT Yoga Short Form A. Hydrate and fuel within 30 minutes. Journal post-training session SOP.

Week 7: De-load Week

Motivation Through Inspiration

When I started the US CrossFit gym in Encinitas, California, I wanted to find out what motivated my clients. Those who came with an extrinsic (external) motivation—like looking better in a bathing suit, being more fit, or shedding the holiday pounds—lasted an average of 3.2 months. Then they disappeared. Their motivation broke the inertia from their prior efforts, but it couldn't accelerate them to the next level.

One day a stray cat walked in named Bobby. He'd been attending meetings for a few months at AA two doors down. Bobby looked like a sickly stick. I figured he wouldn't last a week.

"Bobby, why are you here?"

He smiled. "Been drinkin' and usin' for ten years and almost killed myself. A friend finally hauled me to AA. At meetings I'd see you guys doin' all this crazy stuff. Wondered whether that could be me. So here I am. I wanna feel like a real man."

I'd been wrong to judge him. He'd birthed desire at the bottom he'd hit, one he never wanted to go back to. Bobby struggled but stuck with it. Day in and day out he kept showing up. He worked on his mind-set. He stayed late to work his core and pick up nuggets from me and the coaching staff. His intrinsic (internal) motivation surpassed most all of our clients. Life is full of surprises.

Twelve months later, Bobby won the Fire in the Belly award at Kokoro Camp 12. His speech still makes me proud.

"Where else can you train your heart? . . . This was just an amazing experience. I'm so humbled by you all . . . and very grateful!"

Bobby was a real man. His journey was just beginning.

MOTIVATION THROUGH INSPIRATION LEADS TO long-term commitment. *Inspire* means "to feel the spirit within." *Motivate* means "to move." Move your spirit through your training. That's what Bobby did. He discovered a deep intrinsic motivation to continue. Every time he came to the gym, he connected to his purpose in life—moving from survival to significance as a man.

Breaking the inertia of old habits gets you started. But it must give way to motivation through inspiration. Then you'll train because you love it. The journey will reward your spirit, and you'll keep moving in return.

MONDAY

BASELINE: pre-SOP and box breathing

- ROM drills
- 30–20–10 reps of wall balls, sit-ups

STRENGTH: 10 rounds, every 60 seconds, perform 2x back squats at 65 percent 1 RM

STAMINA: 5 rounds, not timed—5x back squats at 65 percent 1 RM, 20x 4-count mountain climbers, 60-second farmer's carry (55#/35#)

WORK CAPACITY: CrossFit's "Cindy"—AMRAP in 20 minutes of:

- 5x pull-ups
- 10x push-ups
- 15x air squats

DURABILITY: 4-mile timed run (goal is under 30 minutes). 100x 4-count flutter kicks, 100x wave-offs. SEALFIT Yoga Short Form B. Hydrate and fuel within 30 minutes. Journal post-training session SOP.

BASELINE: pre-SOP and box breathing

- ROM drills
- 5 rounds—200m run, 5x strict presses, 5x push presses, 5x jerks, 5x pull-ups (45#/65#/75#)

STRENGTH: 10 rounds, every 60 seconds, perform 2x push presses at 65 percent 1 RM

STAMINA: chipper, not timed—25x push presses at 65 percent 1 RM, 50x ring dips, 400m weighted walking lunge (35#/25#)

WORK CAPACITY: complete 5 RFT of:

- 30x sandbag lunges (60#/40#)
- 15x sandbag cleans (60#/40#)
- 200m row

DURABILITY: 10x 100m sprints (15-second interval). SEALFIT Yoga Short Form A. Hydrate and fuel within 30 minutes. Journal post-training session SOP.

WEDNESDAY [WEEK 7: DE-LOAD WEEK]

BASELINE: pre-SOP and box breathing

- ROM drills
- 20 minutes of grinder PT

ENDURANCE: As time allows, LSD run, bike, swim

DURABILITY: SEALFIT Yoga (any form) or active stretch. Hydrate and fuel within 30 minutes. Journal post-training session SOP.

BASELINE: pre-SOP and box breathing

- ROM drills
- 4 rounds—barbell complex* with push-up chaser (75#–105#)

STRENGTH: 10 rounds, every 60 seconds, perform 2x deadlifts at 65 percent 1 RM

STAMINA: 4 rounds, not timed—5x deadlifts at 65 percent 1 RM, 3x max height box jumps, max time handstand hold

WORK CAPACITY: complete for time:

- 1,000m row
- 50x overhead squats (75#/55#)
- 25x burpees

DURABILITY: 2-mile run with weighted vest. 100x sit-ups, 100x leg levers. SEALFIT Yoga hip mobility drill. Hydrate and fuel within 30 minutes. Journal post-training session SOP.

Note: Barbell complex—with 45# bar (30# women) do 6x deadlifts, 6x bent-over rows, 6x hang power cleans, 6x front squats, 6x push presses, 6x back squats (see www.sealfit.com /videos).

FRIDAY [WEEK 7: DE-LOAD WEEK]

BASELINE: pre-SOP and box breathing

- ROM drills
- 15x sandbag get-ups
- 400m run
- 15x sandbag get-ups

STRENGTH: 10 rounds, every 60 seconds, perform 2x bench presses at 65 percent 1 RM

STAMINA: chipper, not timed—25x bench presses at 65 percent 1 RM, 75x supine ring pull-ups, 800m buddy carry

WORK CAPACITY: "Running Fran"—for time:

- 800m run
- 21–15–9 thrusters (95#/65#), pull-ups
- 800m run

DURABILITY: 1x 500m row sprint. 1x max plank, 1x max wall sit. SEALFIT Yoga Short Form A. Hydrate and fuel within 30 minutes. Journal post-training session SOP.

BASELINE: pre-SOP and box breathing

- ROM drills
- 3 rounds of 50x jump ropes, 25x air squats, 15x push-ups, 5x pull-ups

WORK CAPACITY: "300 Spartans"—for time:

- 25x pull-ups
- 50x deadlifts (135#/95#)
- 50x push-ups
- 50x box jumps (24 or 20 inches)
- 50x floor wipers (135#/95#)
- 50x KB clean and presses (16kg/12kg)
- 25x pull-ups

DURABILITY: 5,000m row. SEALFIT Yoga (any form). Hydrate and fuel within 30 minutes. Journal post-training session SOP.

Week 8: Personal Record Phase

Courage

"When ya headin' back to the playground, Glen?"

Doherty and I were finishing up a conversation about SEALFIT long-term training plans. A former SEAL and one of my top coaches, Glen also happened to be a contractor for the "Agency" and was about to shoot out on a trip to Libya.

"Head out Wednesday," he said. "Hope this'll be my last gig."

"Really?" My voice didn't hide my hope that he would hang it up soon. It was a young man's game. Glen had just turned 40.

"Yeah, gettin' tired of this shit. I really want to settle down and dig into somethin' new."

"Just keep your head down and stay safe," I said, as he walked away. It was the last time I saw him.

I got the text from my friend, Brandon Webb, on September 12, 2012. Glen had been killed in Libya with Ty Woods, another SEAL. I remembered Ty from my early operating days. Brandon and I were devastated. Then the back-channel news rolled in.

Glen and Ty heard gunfire and explosions as they rested in their safe house some distance from the American embassy in Benghazi. They turned on their radio and heard calls for help. Both thought about it for a moment and then jumped in their vehicle, racing to the embassy. Grabbing weapons off fleeing Libyan security guards, they fought their way in and freed eighteen trapped Americans in a 6-hour gunfight. They then left the scene and returned to the safe house. They were followed.

Another 10-hour gunfight ensued. The two warriors eliminated over sixty of the enemy combatants. Finally a mortar ended their last stand. Glen and Ty redefined courage for all warriors on that fateful day. They'll forever be remembered as heroes by those who care to learn the truth.

This story, along with the first about Michael Monsoor, may seem extreme in a book about training. The bottom line is that neither Glen or Michael would have had the honor or courage to act as they did without honing their warrior disciplines through intense training. SEALFIT requires courage to stick with and endure the challenges. Along the way, it cultivates your courage muscle. Taking courageous action will become common. As it did with Glen, it will make you uncommon. Reflect upon the courage of these selfless men this week. Ask yourself how you can meet their standard when called upon.

Good luck, and *hooyah,* Glen and Ty!

MONDAY

BASELINE: pre-SOP and box breathing

- ROM drills
- 500m row
- work up to 1 RM back squat

STRENGTH: back squat—1 rep at −5 percent of 1 RM, 4 sets × 1 rep at −10 percent of 1 RM

STAMINA: 5 rounds, not timed—15x back squats at 35 percent 1 RM, 1x suicide sprint (0m–10m–20m), max time chin above the bar hold

WORK CAPACITY: complete the following for time:

- 1-mile run
- 30x clean and jerks (135#/95#)
- 10x rope ascents

DURABILITY: 4-mile timed run. 40x GHD sit-ups. SEALFIT Yoga Short Form A. Hydrate and fuel within 30 minutes. Journal post-training session SOP.

BASELINE: pre-SOP and box breathing

- ROM drills
- 800m run
- work up to 1 RM push press

STRENGTH: push press—1 rep at −5 percent of 1 RM, 4 sets × 1 rep at −10 percent of 1 RM

STAMINA: chipper, not timed—50x push presses at 35 percent 1 RM, 75x elevated push-ups, 800m farmer's walk (75 percent of body weight)

WORK CAPACITY: complete 10–9–8–7–6–5–4–3–2–1 of:

- thrusters (95#/65#)
- burpees
- box jumps (24 or 20 inches)

DURABILITY: Tabata row. Tabata = 8 rounds of 20 seconds work, 10-second rest. SEALFIT Yoga Short Form B. Hydrate and fuel within 30 minutes. Journal post-training session SOP.

WEDNESDAY [WEEK 8: PERSONAL RECORD PHASE]

BASELINE: pre-SOP and box breathing

- ROM drills
- 20 minutes of grinder PT

ENDURANCE: As time allows, LSD run, bike, swim

DURABILITY: SEALFIT Yoga (any form) or active stretch. Hydrate and fuel within 30 minutes. Journal post-training session SOP.

BASELINE: pre-SOP and box breathing

- ROM drills
- 500m row
- work up to 1 RM deadlift

STRENGTH: deadlift—1 rep at −5 percent of 1 RM, 4 sets × 1 rep at −10 percent of 1 RM

STAMINA: 4 rounds, not timed—20x deadlifts at 35 percent 1 RM, 5x pistols (each leg), 50m bear crawl

WORK CAPACITY: AMRAP in 15 minutes of:

- 15x hang power cleans (95#/65#)
- 15x toes to bars
- 100m sprint

DURABILITY: 2-mile recovery run. 100x 4-count flutter kicks, 100x leg levers. SEALFIT Yoga hip mobility drill. Hydrate and fuel within 30 minutes. Journal post-training session SOP.

FRIDAY [WEEK 8: PERSONAL RECORD PHASE]

BASELINE: pre-SOP and box breathing

- ROM drills
- 800m run
- work up to 1 RM bench press

STRENGTH: bench press—1 rep at −5 percent of 1 RM, 4 sets × 1 rep at −10 percent of 1 RM

STAMINA: chipper, not timed—50x bench presses at 35 percent 1 RM, 75x hand release push-ups, 400m weighted walking lunge (55#/35#)

WORK CAPACITY: complete 5 rounds, each for time:

- 20x KB swings (55#/35#)*
- 30x wall balls (20#/14#)*
- 40x sit-ups*
- 50x steps walking lunge*

DURABILITY: 1x mile sprint. SEALFIT Yoga shoulder mobility drill. Hydrate and fuel within 30 minutes. Journal post-training session SOP.

Note: Rest 2 minutes between each round.

BASELINE: pre-SOP and box breathing

- ROM drills
- 4 rounds: Frog Complex with push-up chaser (Start with 75#/55# and increase load 10# each set until you finish at 105#/85#.)

WORK CAPACITY: baseline #3—for time complete:

- 500m row (substitute a run if you don't have a rower)
- 40x air squats
- 30x sit-ups
- 20x push-ups
- 10x pull-ups

THEN DO MURPH—WITH A WEIGHTED VEST, FOR TIME:

- 1-mile run
- 10 rounds of 10 pull-ups, 20 push-ups, 30 sit-ups
- 1-mile run

DURABILITY: SEALFIT Yoga Short Form A. Hydrate and fuel within 30 minutes. Journal post-training session SOP.

CONGRATULATIONS—

YOU'VE

COMPLETED

THE AOT!

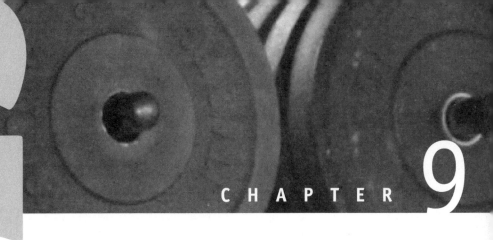

NEEDED: SEALFIT LEADERS

There is no "I" in Team! —BUD/S INSTRUCTOR

BATTLESTAR, YOU'RE A WRECK. THE GUYS ARE IGNORING YOU AND FOLLOWING FUCIARELLI ALREADY. AND FUCH IS THE CLASS LEADING PETTY OFFICER—YOU'RE THE CLASS LEADER, FOR GOD'S SAKE! GET YOUR SHIT TOGETHER AND START LEADING YOUR MEN!"

The proctor of my BUD/S class was reading Battlestar the riot act. Lieutenant Battlestar (an obvious pseudonym that was his actual nickname!) had transplanted himself from the Navy's legal corps to BUD/S. He was class leader by virtue of being the senior officer in the class. All other leadership qualities fell short, it appeared. As a newly minted ensign, I was also just finding my feet as a leader. No one taught me much about leadership before BUD/S, but the lieutenant was supposed to have developed some during his 7 years in the Navy. The schoolhouse of BUD/S required some modicum of leadership prowess as an officer, but nothing compared to what was expected at the team level. I had only a short time span to learn some solid leadership skills—once ordered to a team I would be handed sixteen souls and millions of dollars' worth of equipment. Then 3, 2, 1 . . . go! At least at BUD/S I was getting a backstage pass to see how it is *not* done . . . by observing Battlestar muddle his way through.

The morning after the chat with the proctor, Battlestar had the class lined up 45 minutes early for the timed run. I wasn't happy—every minute of sleep was precious. When the instructors showed up and started orchestrating chaos, he lost control and started running around like a chicken with his head cut off. Fuciarelli stood still and calmly took control of the class. That was the last straw. They fired the lieutenant on the spot and put another officer in charge. Though he graduated BUD/S, I heard that Battlestar had gotten run out of the teams about 2 years later. Leadership is difficult to learn if you don't have the character to lead.

I gleaned from Battlestar's actions what one had to do and be in order to lead well. These included:

- **LEAD FROM THE FRONT.** Be able to perform the basic tasks you're asking others to perform at some level of skill. If the task is overly complex, at a minimum the leader needs to understand the requirements and challenges and be able to communicate them.

- **LEAD WITH HEART.** Don't be in it for yourself; you must actually care for your teammates.

- **LEAD WITH VISION.** Nothing squashes team spirit quicker than an uninspired leader with no vision for how to kick ass and take names. We quickly tuned out Battlestar as he droned instructions to the team.

- **LEAD WITH RISK.** Allow your team to take risks, and share that risk with your team.

You must be first out the door on a jump or first to engage the enemy. They have to come with you. You can't hide behind the paperwork and task from the rear. You can't do it all on your own.

- ■ **LEAD WITH HUMILITY.** A big ego is a big turnoff. Though Battlestar was not boastful, he wasn't humble or self-aware of his limitations. Leading from that place gets people injured or, at the very least, seriously demoralized.

After "learning" leadership lessons compliments of Battlestar, I sought to test my theories out and observe other successful leaders, such as Fuciarelli. It was one thing to see and hear a concept and another completely to put it into play. True leadership seemed to be more character traits than behavioral guidelines. I began to learn how to lead other human beings through trial and error. It was a painful process—though not as painful as Battlestar's was at BUD/S. It continues to this day.

What About You?

Sure, Mark, I want to be a leader. Where do I start?

Good question!

Start where I started—acknowledge that you aren't perfect and that authentic leadership requires you to learn about human behavior first. Study it in yourself and others. Observe and test your learning against reality in a process of trial and error. Open yourself up to the risk of failure . . . there's simply no better way to earn leadership stripes. Fall down seven times. Get up eight! It'll develop the humility you lack. (It did in me!) Over time you'll prove trustworthy to your teammates, and in turn, they'll convey to you the right to lead them. It happens quietly, at a very subtle level. Let's look at a few leadership principles that will help you be an authentic leader and build an elite team.

Eat Your Own Dog Food

You must lead from the front. You simply cannot ask your team to do things you aren't willing or able to do yourself. You don't have to be the best at everything, just willing to *do* your best. Be willing to share their risk and experiences. This forges the team bond at a deep level.

How does this apply to your training? First, though SEALFIT training can be done solo, it's more powerful with a team. If you don't have a team, recruit one. Seriously. Find some people to go through this training with you. Use this experience to forge your leadership skills. When coaching them, *eat the dog food you feed* to the team—meaning train side by side with them. Keep one eye on safety and form and the other on your own training. For this to work well, your teammates must be at a level of physical development such that:

1. They won't hurt themselves.

2. They won't slow the team down.

3. You won't have to spend an inordinate amount of time on skill development or remedial work.

4. They'll be great teammates and a lot of fun!

Don't worry about screwing up. Your team will see you as human. They'll respect you greatly for joining them in risking failure and humiliation. No one wants to be led by an unfeeling robot. Gone are the days when the leader can lord over a team as a demagogue. By the way, the team loves it when the boss can beat them at a workout. You may leave your guts on the floor, but you'll earn points along the way.

Safety Trumps Hard

After grinding my team down at HQ, when I thought all was going well, I learned a new lesson: The universe will slow you down if you don't do it yourself. Executing a burpee box jump, I failed to put my full awareness into the movement. I landed at an angle, spitting the box out from under me. I flew backward, breaking my fall with my wrist. The doctors put me into a cast to lick my wound. I committed to developing more balance and safety in the training.

Safety trumps hard. Balance the training to prevent injuries, and be smart about how you plan to execute the mission. It's easy to grind a teammate into the ground. Not everyone is at the same level. If you strive to meet them where they are, you won't run them ragged. They're not much use if 30 percent sit injured on the bench.

No plan survives first contact with reality—you have to adapt and innovate on the fly. Some tips for a safe training evolution:

1. Have a plan and brief it.

2. Assign roles—assistant leaders, medic, scribe, etc.

3. Prepare equipment and scout location (if new).

4. Check weather, tides, or other "environmental partners."

5. Have a med plan and med kit on site.

6. Deal with injuries right away—veer toward being overcautious at the point of injury, and aggressive in getting the injured teammate back into the game.

7. Debrief the training session and try to do one thing better the next time.

Integrity and Hard Work

In the early days I'd sometimes let the team off the hook on a particularly tough workout. They gladly accepted the gift, but secretly wished that I had pushed them harder. Hard work is a habit. Use it or lose it. Developing that muscle is something the world could use more of—so lead by example. It's your responsibility to hold the team accountable. If they won't put out, call an *all stop* and inspire them to step up their game. Ask them which dog they're feeding. Then feed the courage dog for them!

What if a new teammate cheats on rep count? One time—chalk it up to ignorance. Twice—let the hammer fall. Three times—off the team. Expect absolute integrity at all times. You may cringe at this statement, but subtle public humiliation can be a surefire way to train integrity in an adult. If you push the behavior under the rug or deal with it in private to avoid embarrassment, the lesson will not be painful enough to alter it. (*Note:* Use this sparingly and with discretion.)

Follow these simple rules, and you'll develop a culture of hard work and mutual respect. Just because it's hard doesn't mean it can't be fun. My experience has taught me that hard fun is more rewarding than easy fun. The positive attitude you and the team cultivate leaves no room for caustic remarks or negative behavior. Remember, it takes only one bad apple to spoil the bunch. Forge a warrior mind-set in your team. They'll enjoy the satisfaction and sense of accomplishment that accompanies SEALFIT training. At the finish line, it's the hardest-working team that wins, not necessarily the most talented.

Self-Reliant Leaders

I still train with my HQ team as much as possible. I don't have to direct them to set up gear or prepare for the session . . . it just happens. If I'm not there, someone else takes charge. We start on time with box breathing and then immediately get busy. Though we have a ton of fun, the focus is on the work, not the fun. The fun arrives as a result of the hard work and the team bond that forms. The team takes care of the team first, then the swim buddy, and then themselves last. Because we all understand the set-up, safety, transitions, and the leader's needs, we've become a self-reliant team.

In the SEALs, everyone is a leader and a follower. When my CO was mentoring me, he was leading. Then I turned around and led my platoon on a training mission. During that mission, my dive expert led the dive and my jump expert led the jump. I followed more than I led on those days—standard operating procedure. You must develop *leader*ship and *follower*ship in tandem. How can you lead if you can't follow?

Many of today's leaders are out of touch with the individual and collective realities of their teams. Learning when to step up to lead and when to step back to follow is a milestone for an authentic leader. Set your ego aside. Let others lead for a change. When you are needed again, step up and take charge! If you're an aspiring leader, ask for a shot at leading the team or a squad. You'll be an elite team when you have self-reliant leaders and followers at all levels.

Team Beats Alone

"Take your eyes off yourself and put them on your teammates!" shouts a SEALFIT coach during Kokoro Camp. "Imagine what would happen if every teammate put your needs ahead of theirs? You'll feel supported and more powerful. And of course you'll want to reciprocate!"

The lesson registered, and everyone under the 330-pound log began encouraging and supporting one another. What had just seemed impossible moved by the force of a united team.

That's the magic of true team training. Getting to this place is not as simple as reading these words, though. It often takes us a full 50 hours of nonstop training in Kokoro Camp to get everyone to act with this level of selflessness. But when it happens—*shazam*—performance explodes!

Your shift from selfishness to caring has a powerful, positive effect on your own energy. You simply can't take care of someone else in a negative state. Try it to prove me wrong. It's very difficult. They won't accept your help if you're negative. You have to care with positive energy.

Service also exerts a powerful positive pull on their energy. Caring for another human requires you to connect with the highest of human emotions—love. When love is expressed in action, such as serving another, it pushes out negative thoughts or behavior.

Put your eyes on your teammates by supporting them with encouraging words during rough times and helping them meet their mission. This demonstrates your willingness to understand their world and share their risk, the best form of sharing, even better than sharing your MRE! Sharing risk and experience equally gives you credibility and trust. As trust grows, so does personal accountability. No one wants to let the team down. You share a common bond and become "brothers-in-arms," so to speak.

Research by Dr. Paul Zak, author of *The Moral Molecule*, has shown that a hormone called oxytocin is released when we care for another. Caring is a physiological trigger to the psychological feeling of love. Pretty cool. There's even a scientific explanation to my theory about why team beats alone. (See audio podcast with Dr. Zak [www.sealfit.com/8weeks].)

A team also increases individual responsibility, something lacking in our society. According to the SEAL ethos, you are responsible for your actions *and* those of your teammates. Those are higher stakes than just letting yourself down. The burden is heavy at first, but over time you'll accept it as a new normal. Caring for your team is an enormous responsibility, but guess what? You're not alone.

Let's be clear—it's much easier to be mentally tough when you have a herd of tough guys and girls watching your back. Team training enhances mental toughness, because you're held highly accountable. Every action risks exposure of vulnerability, forcing you to step it up a few notches. Being on a team helps develop a greater awareness, sharpens communication, and enhances problem solving under stress. In essence, through your training you develop your mind and emotions for the rigors of leadership and being a team player. Or you can go back to strolling around a big box gym waiting for the treadmill!

One final comment about team training—it should be a blast. Humor is a hallmark of mental toughness. A team that jokes together stays together. Appoint yourself as head of the Department of Humor. SEAL training had me convinced that the Navy sent the instructors to funny school. They had us laughing while they kicked our butts all over the base. I laughed through 6 months of hell, just as you should laugh through your 8 weeks to SEALFIT training!

You'll never be perfect. Take the risk. Become a SEALFIT leader.

Training Session

Your training session today: Repeat the baseline screening test from chapter 1. Journal your results and report them to me at info@sealfit.com. Congratulations—you've made it!

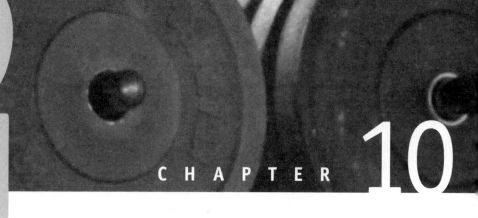

CHAPTER 10

YOU'RE NOT COMMON

The good things of prosperity are to be wished; but the good things that belong to adversity are to be admired. —SENECA

WHAT'S GOING ON, VIN? WHY AREN'T YOU OUT THERE DANCING AND HOOTING IT UP WITH YOUR BROTHERS?"

"DON'T FEEL LIKE IT, DAD. I HATE MY JOB. I'M NOT HAPPY."

There, he said it. His life basically sucked, and he had everything he needed. He had a family. Both parents were together. He'd gone to a great college and had an enviable job. Why did he feel so empty, so vacant? Everyone else seemed happy, able to let go and have fun. He felt totally closed, shut down, encased in an emotional casket.

On the train back to New York the next day, Vin resolved to make a change. He hated his job, even though he'd taken it for all the right reasons, he thought. The money was great. It had prestige. More important, the experience, along with the MBA and CPA, laid an excellent foundation for a future in the family business. But who was he doing it for—his family, his society, or himself? The answer became clear in that moment . . . he wasn't living his own life.

In that instant, Vin felt a shift to a new layer of self-awareness as a lightening of the load. The stress of living his life for someone else's values gave way to a new energy, a cautious excitement over the possibilities that lay ahead. *I'm going to start going to those meditation classes on Thursday nights*, he thought to himself. *That'll help me get clear about what to do, where to go.*

As he drifted off to sleep, he fantasized about being on a grand adventure far from home, facing great challenges, and overcoming the obstacles with ease. He was a master swordsman who slew his enemies with ease, yet was a humble and graceful man. *Someday*, he thought, *someday that will be me.*

TWENTY-FIVE YEARS LATER, AN OLDER Vin stepped up to the lectern. Though weathered a bit by the years, he was eminently fit. A fire burned bright in his eyes. He scanned the audience, who were there to learn from him. Not completely comfortable speaking in front of a crowd, he turned away for a moment and asked the Great Spirit to speak through him, to inspire this next generation of warriors. Then he smiled and asked, "Why are you here?"

"We're here to learn and train," the crowd said, puzzled.

"I know you're here to learn and train. But why are you really *here*? On this planet . . . What's your purpose? We all have a unique reason for being here, and it's critical that you find out what it is, this weekend!"

The faces revealed both concern and, in some, a knowing.

"If you can't figure it out, you won't make it through the fire. Discovering your 'why' is like taking a big drink from the well after walking across the Sahara Desert. It feels like coming home.

"As a young man I had it all, but was unhappy in spite of it. I felt lost, as if I were marking time. I tried working out harder and longer. I tried making more money, traveling, and women. The emptiness grew. When the pain of my situation got so acute that I couldn't handle the self-imposed isolation, I stumbled into a martial arts dojo and met my future mentor, a real-life Miyamato Musashi. Remembering my fantasy of the master swordsman, I signed up, thinking it might help.

"It did, but in a way I could never have expected. Grinding my character down on the gritty training floor was followed by polishing it in the serene meditation hall. Slowly and methodically I tuned my body, mind, emotions, and intuition to a new vibration—one that allowed me to hear my inner voice. That voice told me I wasn't living my purpose, that my misery would endure until I could align with my purpose.

"I found the inspiration to change in that place long ago. It took me through the hell of Navy SEAL training. I emerged as the honor graduate. I learned humility through constant screwups and patient mentors who forced me to shed my immaturity. I found courage in the teammates who served, bled, and sometimes died alongside me. No part of it came easy. My journey continues to this day, through SEALFIT."

Five Stages from Common to Extraordinary

I'm Vin (as in Mark Di"vin"e). I'm not much different than you. I've been on life's roller coaster with extreme highs and dismal lows. Misdiagnosed with melanoma and given 6 months to live at 17, I look back at my formative years with wonder how I made it this far. I'm so grateful that I found a mentor to steer me toward my purpose. The alternative is hard to imagine. I was an arrogant teen, thinking I stood on top of the world. Unconscious incompetence ruled me, a stage I call *Ignorance*—lasting from childhood into my early 20s. Many people go through their whole lives at this level of development. Woe is them.

The blowback of reality hit me as I entered the workforce. I had to wake up quickly. I needed many skills that weren't taught or passed down to me. Perhaps you are or were in the same boat. Why aren't they taught? Why would we send our young men and women out into the world with no deep skills concerning how to live well? Curious. Regardless, there I was, seeking skills and knowledge to help me navigate the internal and external mines I stepped on.

My mentor appeared at that precise moment when he was most needed. I stepped out into the next stage of my journey, one of conscious incompetence. During this next stage, I developed an internal sense of my purpose, passion, and principles, and then worked to align these through a new career in the SEALs. I spent a lot of time seeking truth about the way the world and humans operated. I call this stage of my growth *self-awareness*—lasting from my early 20s until my early 30s.

As my training took root, something magical started to happen. I developed greater and greater control over my thoughts, emotions, and body. The growth I experienced accelerated, fueled by the integrated training I was doing, including yoga, martial arts, Navy SEAL–style physical training, and a lot of reading and study. During this stage I moved from conscious incompetence to conscious competence. My actions became more confident and focused. I began an entrepreneurial career after the SEALs. In spite of stubbed toes, I saw success and happiness accruing. I began to move from seeking truth to experiencing a wisdom that comes from deeper awareness of others and the systems I operated in. I knew I couldn't go it alone, that a team in synch was a magical thing. I call this stage *self-control*—lasting from my early 30s until mid-40s.

The fourth major stage of my developmental journey is still a work in progress. I've moved from conscious competence to an unconscious competence in many actions and areas of my life. Right action will often flow out of me with little or no active thought. When I try to muscle my way through things I get worse results than if I let go and flow with it. I feel a sense of order in the chaos, and have submitted to simplicity, humility, and the value of all life. This stage is felt as love informed by wisdom and truth. I call it *self-mastery*.

I have occasional glimpses of another stage unfolding rapidly that I can only describe as *blissful flow*. I believe this is the same as the Apache concept of sacred silence, or the Japanese concept of *shibumi*—effortless perfection. It's when a self-mastered individual yokes his or her ego with spirit in a blissful union, leading to peace, harmony, and joy. I'm not actively seeking this prize. I expect it can be attained only by embracing each moment of the journey with enthusiasm. My training plan is the framework for that journey, as is yours for your own journey.

You may find similarities between my stages of development and your own. I offered them as reference points, like trail markers on a mountain trail. They closely follow the psychological development models of transpersonal psychology and integral theory, though the terms are different (and my focus in this book is on performance versus consciousness itself). Along the way you'll need to eradicate hate, harness your fears, and cultivate love for yourself and your teammates.

Love, Fear, and Hate

Love and fear are the only two emotions that emerge with us from the womb. All other emotions evolve from these two. Fear only has three true manifestations:

- fear of being alone
- fear of being unworthy
- fear of being unsafe

It's not hard to see why a child would act out of fear of these three. It *is* hard to see why a mature adult would continue to act out in mutated, immature aspects of these. Fear of being alone causes clinging and control to ensure certainty, and this always leads to the pushing away of others and being alone. Fear of being unworthy causes one to show the opposite, and be boastful and loud, in a need to be seen and feel significant. Again it yields the opposite results. Fear of being unsafe leads to a cloistered, unadventurous life, the most unsafe life to live. Predators feed off this energy and know exactly who to target.

No doubt fear has a place in the survival of humans and is hard-coded into our DNA. Our ancestors rightly feared the neighboring tribe that was literally out to kill them and take their food and women. In modern times it's right to fear the intruder in your home. Fear activates our defense mechanisms. It allows us to take more powerful action. However, it must be understood, controlled, and used to our advantage. Fear management occurs as a result of developing courage through your SEALFIT training. Other ways to develop it include martial arts, contact sports, and living close to the earth where survival relies on controlling fear.

A healthy approach to learning about the three fears would have you face the fear and replace it with courage. Courage is a stepping-stone to love. So:

- Replace fear of being alone with the courage to learn intimacy.
- Replace fear of being unworthy with the courage to serve others and to be worthy of their love.
- Replace fear of being unsafe with the courage to learn to defend yourself.

What about love? As you move toward self-mastery—gaining self-awareness and self-control—you'll naturally begin to experience more love in your life. Could we say that love is in contrast to those things we most fear?

- **Love of being safe.**
- **Love of feeling worthy.**
- **Love of being intimately connected.**

This doesn't feel right to me. We certainly desire those to exist in contrast to the three fears, but love is an entirely different energy. The absence of fear is not love, but courage. The absence of love is not fear, but emptiness. Love blooms only in relationship.

And finally, what about hate? Hate sucks, that's what. Hate is when all three fears exist in the same space and time, in their most mutated form. To hate another is to hate yourself and all of life. This stanza from a poem written in 1807 by Shadow Walker, an Apache scout, expresses his struggle with the warrior's dilemma—how to take a life if you honor all life:

> *Forgive me, Grandfather, for now I must pick up the lance. Direct my mind, direct my heart, so that there is no hatred, rage, or revenge.*

Even when we have so-called enemies, we can act out of love for them, not hate. Our world will be a different place when all of us learn this truth. I ask again, *Why are you here?* Why are you reading this book? What are you going to do if you find you're not living your purpose? What if you still operate from fear or experience hate? Why the heck are we talking about this in a book about training?

Training IS Life

You could say, "There's a lot more to life than training." That would be true, to some. Or you could say, "Training is life!" This would also be true, for some. Which do you think will lead to mastery and flow? You know the answer. Look at training as your teammate in human alchemy, driving you relentlessly toward your highest potential as a human. You'll evolve through your training. I will mentor you, if you allow me to. The concepts, tools, and practices introduced alongside the physical training in this book will light up your journey as you move from self-awareness to self-control to self-mastery and then to blissful flow. Along the way you will be:

1. Finding your purpose and aligning with it.

2. Learning to plan and set proper goals.

3. Developing an ethical foundation for excellence.

4. Forging physical, mental, and emotional resiliency.

5. Working "in" while working out—using immersion in the moment, vivid visualization, and sensory development to deepen personal awareness and intuition in your daily actions.

6. Controlling your breath for optimal performance—turning eustress into success.

7. Developing deep powers of concentration on a single task, so that you can accomplish anything worthy you set out for yourself.

8. Developing authenticity as a teammate and leader.

9. Finding flow in all you do—your training, performing, and just being.

Sounds uncommon, doesn't it? It does, because it is. Common is doing the same thing every day and expecting different results. Common is living a life for someone else's needs. Common is being blind to your unique purpose and contribution to the world. Common is shying from challenge, shirking responsibility, and falling back in the face of defeat. Common is judging, bickering, sneering, gossiping, and belittling others. Common is expecting things to be given to you, rather than embracing the joy of hard work. Common is living a life of regret, rather than suffering the pain of discipline.

But that doesn't sound like you. It isn't, or you wouldn't have read this far. Whether you've finished the training in this book, or are about to start, you must remember this:

YOU'RE NOT COMMON!
YOU'RE SEALFIT.

God bless you. I wish you fair winds and following seas. *Hooyah!*

Unbeatable Mind Power Resources

1. The Unbeatable Mind Stand

1. The world is *Chaotic* and *Dangerous*.

2. Destiny favors the prepared in *Mind*, *Body*, and *Spirit*.

3. Personal growth must encompass the *Whole Person* and be *Integrated* to accelerate growth.

4. There is an *Athlete* and a *Warrior* within everyone. We differ only in degree and purpose.

5. Leadership is shown through *Example* and cultivated in the *Arena*.

6. True learning is *Experiential* and the best learning is through *Trial* and *Error*. We use what works and discard what doesn't.

7. We treat others with *Respect*, *Compassion*, and, if necessary, *Tough Love*.

8. To qualify for the team you must have a burning desire to do *Better Every Day*, to meet your *Commitments*, and to maintain a *Winning Attitude*.

2. The Three Ps

Know the other and know the self, in a hundred battles you will be victorious; know the self but not the other, in a hundred battles you will lose half. Know neither the self nor the other, in a hundred battles you will lose all. —SUN TZU

PURPOSE

What is it that you are really supposed to do with your life? What one thing would you focus on if you had nothing holding you back?

PASSION

Who are you? What makes you feel as if your hair is on fire? This informs your purpose when intersected with your skills and talents.

PRINCIPLES

What is it that you truly value? How can you "habituate" these values until you own them?

3. The Morning Ritual

The goal of the morning ritual is to engage your body and mind in a positive manner. You will connect to your purpose, cultivate your optimism and positivity, and ensure that your next actions of the day move the dial toward your goals. We want to energize your physiology and psychology for optimal performance!

STEP 1: Drink a large glass of water, then, sitting comfortably with your journal, ask yourself these empowering questions:

- What and whom am I grateful for today? (Write down what comes up. Cultivate an attitude of gratitude!)
- What am I excited about and looking forward to doing today?
- What is my purpose and do my plans for today connect me to it?
- What can I do to move the dial toward my purpose goals today?
- Who can I reach out to and serve or thank today?

Review your goals and ensure they are still aligned with your purpose.

STEP 2: Morning practice. Set up your space and settle into your morning practice.

- Box breathing practice; 5 minutes.

- SEALFIT Yoga: 10–45 minutes (you can substitute Qi Gong, a light workout, or a brisk walk here).

- From resting pose after your movement conduct a short breath awareness meditation: 5 minutes.

- Visualization or guided visualization: 5 minutes.

- Shower up and get ready for your day.

- Drink another glass of fresh water, and eat a healthy Paleo breakfast.

STEP 3: Before you leave for work, review your daily schedule. Make any adjustments and block time for key project work and your physical training. When you get to your place of work, start performing and don't let others take you off task, off focus, or off purpose. Use your presence practices to stay focused and energized throughout the day. Avoid food and drink that steals your energy (junk food, candy, excessive coffee, Rockstars, 5-hour energy drinks, etc.).

4. The Evening Ritual

Before you settle in for the night, find some quiet space and with your journal perform a "look back" review of your day, from start to finish. Note whether you were on and in the zone today or off and unbalanced. If you note "off," then ask yourself: *Why?* Lack of sleep, diet, a relationship, stress? Then ask yourself what were the top three positive things you accomplished or that happened to you today? Then ask yourself if there are any unresolved issues or questions. Also review your major goals. Pay attention to your dreams and any waking thoughts—the answer will usually be there for you.

5. The Pre-Event (Pretraining) SOP

Use this ritual when facing a major mission, race, or challenge and you simply must be at your peak. Once habituated this can be a 5-minute exercise with a powerful impact on your performance.

- Eliminate external distractions.

- Perform a dirt dive visualization to "size up" your performance in the event and "size down" the opponents or enemy.

- Next, review your goals and your strategy for the mission or challenge.

- Finally, initiate the *Performance Anchor* process. See, feel, and hear your ideal performance state, and start an internal dialogue with a powerful mantra to maintain a positive mind-set, speech, posture, and state of being as you finish your pre-event ritual and launch into performing. Your Performance Anchor should include deep breath control exercises. Elite athletes and Navy SEALs utilize breath control to prepare for missions and events, and so should you. The act of psyching yourself up physically and mentally includes deep diaphragmatic breathing, forced exhalation breaths, combined with powerful visualization and positive affirmations. The breathing doesn't need to be fancy or esoteric—simple, long inhale holds followed by a powerful forced exhale and short exhale hold will do the trick. Repeat it 20x while performing your visualization.

6. The Post-Event (Post-Training) SOP

- *Remember* who helped you along the way by asking yourself gratitude questions. You have survived or accomplished something big, so who can you thank and be grateful for?

- *Reflect* on your performance. How did you do? What did you learn? Did you move the dial on your twenty goals? How can you improve and do even better next time? Was the event worth the time and energy? Would you do it again?

- *Reframe* with a positive lesson: What did you learn? What was the silver lining? Why did it have to happen the way it did?

- *Redirect* your attention to a new mission or challenge.

- *Reengage* your planning and training.

- *Reward* yourself with something simple and meaningful.

7. Goal Setting

Goal setting is simply a process for organizing our focus on achievement of desired results in a systematic and effective manner over a specific time period.

SMART GOALS

- Specific, Measurable, Achievable, Realistic (but Challenging), and Time-bound.

- Long- and short-term—the harder the challenge, the more short-term the goals (in Hell Week they may be "micro-goals" such as making it to the next meal).
- Write your goals down in positive language.
- Develop a strategy for following through on goals.

WHY DOES GOAL SETTING WORK?

- It directs attention to important elements of a skill or process. Focuses us on one vs. many things.
- It mobilizes our efforts in a forward and positive direction (i.e., rudder of a ship).
- It enhances and prolongs persistent effort—keep trying until you make it.
- It fosters development of new strategies for learning and developing.

PITFALLS TO GOAL SETTING

- Fuzzy goals (not specific).
- Too many goals (unrealistic).
- Too short of a time frame (unrealistic).
- Inflexible goals (not achievable—need to flex and mold to reality).
- Lack of process goals—need to work on self while you work on things.
- No follow-up or evaluation of progress—need to check your progress and be held accountable

EXERCISE: Write out top three goals for your personal and professional life. For example: *I will complete 20 perfect consecutive double unders in less than 1 minute by June 30.*

8. Visualization Revisited

MENTAL PROJECTION: Concentrate on and visualize your personal victory. Thereby you create or re-create the desired experience in your mind.

MENTAL REHEARSAL: Practice in your mind's eye. It can be *internal* (from one's own vantage point) or *external* (view self from the perspective of others).

USES: improve concentration; build confidence; control emotions; practice a technical skill; practice a strategy; cope with pain, injury, or cold.

When envisioned well, when you perform the event in "real time" it is not the first time, but one of many times that your mind has done it perfectly before.

Envisioning is like visualization on steroids. It uses ALL your senses. See yourself performing; sense your movement, emotions; hear the sounds of success; feel the actual air, water, handshake, etc.; and smell your environment. Create the experience as close as possible to actual experience, but manipulating the images for perfect results. Include positive thoughts and emotions to burn the image into your subconscious.

- 90 percent of Olympic athletes use visualization, and 97 percent of them claim it helped their performance.

- 94 percent of Olympic coaches use visualization for training, and 100 percent claim it enhances performance.

WHY DOES IT WORK?

Visualized events, if vivid and empowered with emotion, stimulate and program your nervous and muscular system as if you are actually practicing. Additionally, envisioning improves your ability to concentrate, which helps with confidence and stress management.

WHEN TO USE THESE TACTICS

- PRE-EVENT: Goal setting and visualization are primary. Self-talk and arousal control help with training and preparation, and pre-event jitters.

- DURING EVENT: Self-talk and arousal control are primary. Short-term goal setting is secondary.

- POST-EVENT: Self-talk (reframing) and goal setting (modifying and setting new goals) are primary.

Basic Training Program

This program is anything but basic compared to most programs. However, Basic Underwater Demolition SEAL (BUD/S) training is also anything but basic, too, so don't let the word *basic* fool you!

This intermediate workout program will either serve as your final training program or prepare you for the Advanced Operator Training (AOT). If you intend to move on to AOT, running through this program once or twice may be enough. The key is in building capacity for the weight loads and volume. If you can't handle those in this program, you're not ready for AOT. Additionally for Masters—those 45 years or older—the loads in this program may be more appropriate than those in AOT. Busy professionals have a difficult time finding the time for AOT, and that's okay. Remember, I originally built AOT for special operators, though men and women from all walks of life have validated its effectiveness.

BASELINE: pre-SOP and box breathing

- ROM drills—10 minutes
- 3 rounds—250m row, 5x air squats, 5x back squats (45#), 5x push-ups, 30-second plank
- warm up to 65 percent of your 1 RM back squat

STRENGTH: back squat—3 reps × 10 sets at 65 percent 1 RM

WORK CAPACITY: complete the following for time:

- 100x double unders (or substitute 300 singles)
- 80x air squats
- 60x sit-ups
- 40x wall balls (20# men /12# women)
- 20x chest-to-bar pull-ups
- 10x clapping push-ups

DURABILITY: 3 rounds—15x GHD sit-ups, 30-second handstand hold, 10x back extensions. SEALFIT Yoga Short Form A. Hydrate and fuel within 30 minutes. Journal post-training session SOP.

TUESDAY [WEEK 1: BASIC TRAINING PROGRAM]

BASELINE: pre-SOP and box breathing

- ROM drills
- 400m run
- 15x overhead squats (45#/35#)
- 400m run
- 15x kipping pull-ups

WORK CAPACITY: complete 10–9–8–7–6–5–4–3–2–1 of:

- overhead squats (95#/65#)
- ring dips
- lateral jumps over the bar 2x

DURABILITY: 10 rounds—30-second max distance row, 30-second rest (goal is 125m–150m each round). SEALFIT Yoga hip mobility drill. Hydrate and fuel within 30 minutes. Journal post-training session SOP.

KIPPING PULL-UPS

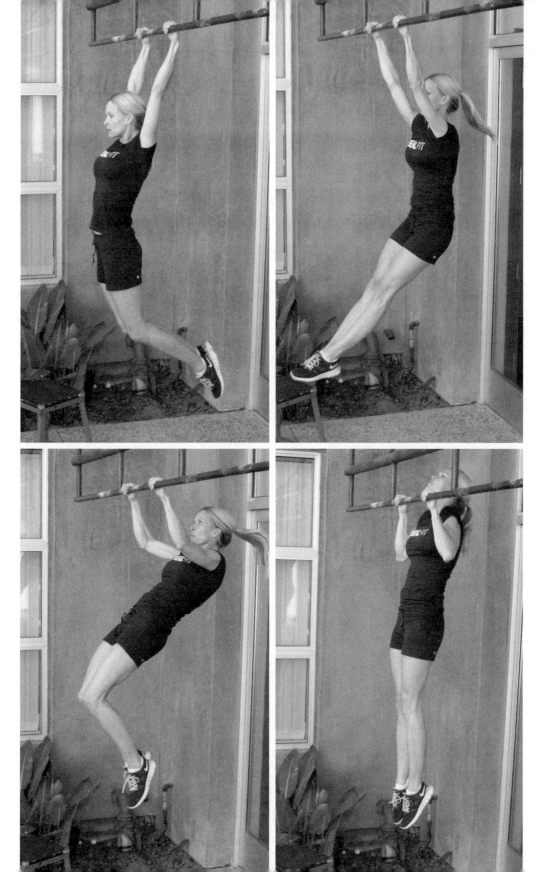

WEDNESDAY [WEEK 1: BASIC TRAINING PROGRAM]

BASELINE: pre-SOP and box breathing

- ROM drills
- 400m run
- 3 rounds—5x strict presses, 5x push presses, 5x push jerks, 10x air squats
- warm up to 65 percent of your 1 RM push press

STRENGTH: push press—3 reps × 10 sets at 65 percent 1 RM

WORK CAPACITY: "AMRAP-athon"—AMRAP in 5 minutes each of:

- 5x box jumps (24 or 20 inches), 7x TTBs (toes to bars)*
- 5x handstand push-ups, 7x wall balls (20#/12#)*
- 5x burpees, 7x DB thrusters (25#/15#)*

DURABILITY: 100x sit-ups, 50x wave-offs (from grinder PT). SEALFIT Yoga Short Form B. Hydrate and fuel within 30 minutes. Journal post-training session SOP.

Note: 1-minute rest between each AMRAP.

BASELINE: pre-SOP and box breathing

- ROM drills
- 20 minutes of grinder PT

ENDURANCE: As time allows, LSD run, bike, swim, row. Distance depends upon your time and endurance level. This is an active recovery endurance session so you can substitute any sport or activity such as a yoga class or long walk.

DURABILITY: Active stretch. Hydrate and fuel within 30 minutes. Journal post-training SOP.

FRIDAY [WEEK 1: BASIC TRAINING PROGRAM]

BASELINE: pre-SOP and box breathing

- ROM drills
- 3 rounds—barbell complex* with push-up chaser (45#/65#)
- warm up to 65 percent of your 1 RM deadlift

STRENGTH: deadlift—3 reps × 10 sets at 65 percent 1 RM

WORK CAPACITY: complete 5 RFT of:

- 5x power cleans (95#–115#/65#–85#)
- 10x push-ups
- 25x double unders

DURABILITY: 30x evil wheels (use a barbell for these if you do not have an evil wheel). SEALFIT Yoga Short Form A. Hydrate and fuel within 30 minutes. Journal post-training session SOP.

Note: Barbell complex—with 45# bar (30# women) do 6x deadlifts, 6x bent-over rows, 6x hang power cleans, 6x front squats, 6x push presses, 6x back squats (see www.sealfit.com /videos).

BASELINE: pre-SOP and box breathing

- ROM drills
- 30–20–10 reps of air squats, KB swings (16kg/12kg)

WORK CAPACITY: 7 rounds, every 2 minutes do:

- 200m run*
- max rep burpees*

DURABILITY: 2 rounds—sprint 400m, jog 400m. SEALFIT Yoga Short Form B or active stretch. Hydrate and fuel within 30 minutes. Journal post-training session SOP. Sunday is a rest day—enjoy!

Note: 1-minute rest between rounds, and score is number of burpees.

MONDAY

BASELINE: pre-SOP and box breathing

- ROM drills
- 500m row
- 15x air squats
- 500m row
- 15x back squats (45#)
- warm up to 70 percent of your 1 RM back squat

STRENGTH: back squat—3 reps × 10 sets at 70 percent 1 RM

WORK CAPACITY: complete 5 RFT of:

- 30x sit-ups
- 20x KB swings (24kg/16kg)
- 10x box jumps (24 or 20 inches)

DURABILITY: 3 rounds—60-second plank, 10x reverse hyperextensions (2/1 x 45# plate). SEALFIT Yoga hip mobility drill. Hydrate and fuel within 30 minutes. Journal post-training session SOP.

BASELINE: pre-SOP and box breathing

- ROM drills
- 3 rounds—3x hang power snatches, 3x overhead squats, 3x snatches, 5x push-ups (45#–65#), 10m bear crawl

WORK CAPACITY: CrossFit's "Snatch Ladder"—every 30 seconds, perform 1x snatch. Increase the weight 10# each round. Men start at 65#, women at 45#. Once you're unable to perform a rep at the required weight, complete 100x double unders as fast as possible.

DURABILITY: 2,000m row as fast as possible (or substitute a 1-mile running sprint). SEALFIT Yoga shoulder mobility drill. Hydrate and fuel within 30 minutes. Journal post-training session SOP.

WEDNESDAY [WEEK 2: BASIC TRAINING PROGRAM]

BASELINE: pre-SOP and box breathing

- ROM drills
- 3 rounds—200m run, 5x push presses (45#), 5x handstand push-ups, 5x pull-ups, 5x PVC shoulder dislocates
- warm up to 70 percent of your 1 RM push press

STRENGTH: push press—3 reps × 10 sets at 70 percent 1 RM

WORK CAPACITY: AMRAP in 15 minutes of:

- 20x ball slams (20#/12#)
- 20x step-ups (20 inch)
- 200m run

DURABILITY: 50x weighted sit-ups (25#/15#), 30x barbell good mornings (45#). SEALFIT Yoga Short Form A. Hydrate and fuel within 30 minutes. Journal post-training session SOP.

BASELINE: pre-SOP and box breathing

- ROM drills
- 20 minutes of grinder PT

ENDURANCE: As time allows, LSD run, bike, swim, row

DURABILITY: SEALFIT Yoga Short Form B. Hydrate and fuel within 30 minutes. Journal post-training session SOP.

FRIDAY [WEEK 2: BASIC TRAINING PROGRAM]

BASELINE: pre-SOP and box breathing

- ROM drills
- 500m row
- 3 rounds—10x KB SDHP (16kg/12kg), 10x push-ups, 10x sit-ups
- warm up to 70 percent of your 1 RM deadlift

STRENGTH: deadlift—3 reps × 10 sets at 70 percent 1 RM

WORK CAPACITY: complete the following for time:

- 150x DB thrusters (35#/25#)

DURABILITY: 3 rounds—20x GHD sit-ups, 10x weighted back extensions (25#/15#). SEALFIT Yoga hip and shoulder mobility drills. Hydrate and fuel within 30 minutes. Journal post-training session SOP.

BASELINE: pre-SOP and box breathing

- ROM drills
- 200m run
- 15x sandbag cleans (40#/30#)
- 200m run
- 15x sandbag cleans (40#/30#)

WORK CAPACITY: 5 rounds—AMRAP in 3 minutes each of:

- 3x power cleans (95#–115#/65#–85#)*
- 6x burpees*
- 9x sit-ups*

DURABILITY: 3-mile run at a moderate pace. SEALFIT Yoga Short Form A. Hydrate and fuel within 30 minutes. Journal post-training session SOP.

Note: 1-minute rest between each AMRAP.

MONDAY

BASELINE: pre-SOP and box breathing

- ROM drills
- 400m run
- 3 rounds—10x air squats, 10x back squats (45#), 10x air squats, groin stretch
- warm up to 75 percent of your 1 RM back squat

STRENGTH: back squat—3 reps × 10 sets at 75 percent 1 RM

WORK CAPACITY: complete 2 RFT of:

- 50x pull-ups
- 75x sit-ups
- 50x overhead squats (75#/45#)
- 75x double unders

DURABILITY: 3 rounds—50x 4-count flutter kicks, 50x leg levers. SEALFIT Yoga Short Form B. Hydrate and fuel within 30 minutes. Journal post-training session SOP.

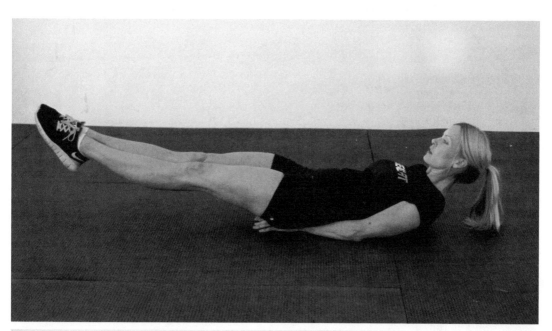

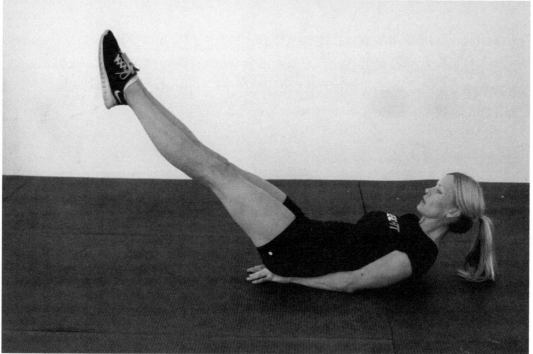

LEG LEVERS

TUESDAY [WEEK 3: BASIC TRAINING PROGRAM]

BASELINE: pre-SOP and box breathing

- ROM drills
- 3 rounds of 250m row
- 5x hang power cleans, 5x front squats, 5x jerks, 5x push-ups. Start at 45#/#25, increase 10# each round

WORK CAPACITY: complete the following for time:

- 800m run
- 15x clean and jerks (105#–135#/75#–95#)
- 800m run

DURABILITY: Tabata row (goal is over 1,000m for men and 800m for women). Tabata = 8 rounds of 20 seconds work, 10-second rest. SEALFIT Yoga Short Form A. Hydrate and fuel within 30 minutes. Journal post-training session SOP.

BASELINE: pre-SOP and box breathing

- ROM drills
- 400m run
- 3 rounds—5x handstand push-ups, 10x push-ups, 60-second jump rope
- warm up to 75 percent of your 1 RM push press

STRENGTH: push press—3 reps × 10 sets at 75 percent 1 RM

WORK CAPACITY: AMRAP in 20 minutes of:

- 3x TGU (Turkish get-ups) each arm (16kg/12kg) (see www.sealfit.com/videos)
- 5x clapping push-ups
- 7x supine ring rows
- 100m sprint

DURABILITY: 50x leg levers, 50x sit-ups. SEALFIT Yoga shoulder mobility drill. Hydrate and fuel within 30 minutes. Journal post-training session SOP.

THURSDAY [WEEK 3: BASIC TRAINING PROGRAM]

BASELINE: pre-SOP and box breathing

- ROM drills
- 20 minutes of grinder PT

ENDURANCE: As time allows, LSD run, bike, swim, row

DURABILITY: SEALFIT Yoga Short Form A or active stretch. Hydrate and fuel within 30 minutes. Journal post-training session SOP.

BASELINE: pre-SOP and box breathing

- ROM drills
- 3 rounds—barbell complex with burpee chaser (45#–65#)
- warm up to 75 percent of your 1 RM deadlift

STRENGTH: deadlift—3 reps × 10 sets at 75 percent 1 RM

WORK CAPACITY: complete 4 RFT of:

- 20x weighted lunges with bar in the racked position (95#/65#)
- 10x hang power snatches (95#/65#)
- 5x snatch grip push presses (95#/65#)

DURABILITY: 3 rounds—1 minute plank hold, 50x sit-ups, 25x wave-offs. SEALFIT Yoga shoulder mobility drill. Hydrate and fuel within 30 minutes. Journal post-training session SOP.

SATURDAY [WEEK 3: BASIC TRAINING PROGRAM]

BASELINE: pre-SOP and box breathing

- ROM drills
- 3 rounds—200m run, 5x jumping pull-ups, 5x dips, 5x jumping squats

WORK CAPACITY: AMRAP in 20 minutes of:

- 5x pull-ups*
- 10x push-ups*
- 15x air squats*

DURABILITY: 800m sprint, 400m sprint, 200m sprint, 100m sprint (1:1 work-to-rest ratio). SEALFIT Yoga Short Form A. Hydrate and fuel within 30 minutes. Journal post-training session SOP.

Note: At 5, 10, and 15 minutes, stop what you are doing and perform 5x burpees.

BASELINE: pre-SOP and box breathing

- ROM drills
- 30–20–10 reps of 4-count mountain climbers, sit-ups
- warm up to 80 percent of your 1 RM back squat

STRENGTH: back squat—3 reps × 10 sets at 80 percent 1 RM

WORK CAPACITY: complete 10–8–6–4–2 reps of:

- Man Makers (35#/25#)
- box jumps (24 or 20 inches)
- toes to bars

DURABILITY: 50x 4-count flutter kicks. 30x reverse hyperextensions (2/1 × 45# plates). SEALFIT Yoga Short Form B. Hydrate and fuel within 30 minutes. Journal post-training session SOP.

TUESDAY [WEEK 4: BASIC TRAINING PROGRAM]

BASELINE: pre-SOP and box breathing

- ROM drills
- 500m row, 5 rounds—3x power cleans, 3x front squats, 3x push jerks, 3x pull-ups (45#–85# men and 25#–65# women)

WORK CAPACITY: complete 3 RFT of:

- 10x ground to overhead (95#/65#)*
- 200m shuttle sprint (50m there and back twice)

DURABILITY: 3 rounds—500m row sprint (2-minute rest between efforts). SEALFIT Yoga Short Form B. Hydrate and fuel within 30 minutes. Journal post-training session SOP.

*Note: Ground to overhead: Get the bar overhead as fast and safely as you can—snatch, clean and jerk, or power clean to push press.

BASELINE: pre-SOP and box breathing

- ROM drills
- 400m run, 15x hand release push-ups
- 400m run, 15x push presses (65#/45#)
- warm up to 80 percent of your 1 RM push press

STRENGTH: push press—3 reps × 10 sets at 80 percent 1 RM

WORK CAPACITY: complete the following for time:

- 5x muscle-ups (substitute 3x ring pull-ups and 3x ring dips if you can't do a muscle-up)
- 50x double unders
- 4x muscle-ups
- 40x double unders
- 3x muscle-ups
- 30x double unders
- 2x muscle-ups
- 20x double unders
- 1x muscle-up
- 10x double unders

DURABILITY: 1-mile recovery run. SEALFIT Yoga shoulder mobility drill. Hydrate and fuel within 30 minutes. Journal post-training session SOP.

THURSDAY [WEEK 4: BASIC TRAINING PROGRAM]

BASELINE: pre-SOP and box breathing

- ROM drills
- 20 minutes of grinder PT

ENDURANCE: As time allows, LSD run, bike, swim, row

DURABILITY: SEALFIT Yoga (any form of active recovery). Hydrate and fuel within 30 minutes. Journal post-training session SOP.

BASELINE: pre-SOP and box breathing

- ROM drills
- 500m row
- 3 rounds—10x SDHP (75#/45#), 10x push-ups, 10x sit-ups
- warm up to 80 percent of your 1 RM deadlift

STRENGTH: deadlift—3 reps × 10 sets at 80 percent 1 RM

WORK CAPACITY: perform in 10 minutes:

- 800m run
- 30x handstand push-ups
- in the remaining time, perform as many double unders as possible

DURABILITY: 100x sit-ups, 100x supermans. SEALFIT Yoga shoulder mobility drill. Hydrate and fuel within 30 minutes. Journal post-training session SOP.

SATURDAY [WEEK 4: BASIC TRAINING PROGRAM]

BASELINE: pre-SOP and box breathing

- ROM drills
- 30–20–10 reps of KB swings (16kg/12kg), air squats, sit-ups

WORK CAPACITY: baseline #2—for time complete:

- 500m row (if you do not have a rower, substitute a run)
- 40x air squats
- 30x sit-ups
- 20x push-ups
- 10x pull-ups

21–15–9 OF:

- thrusters (95#/65#)
- pull-ups

DURABILITY: 8x 200m hill sprints—rest as you walk back down the hill. If you don't have access to a hill, substitute 200m sprints at a 30-second interval. SEALFIT Yoga Short Form B. Hydrate and fuel within 30 minutes. Journal post-training session SOP.

Shopping List

Meat

Protein sources include meat and poultry for meat eaters. Vegetarians must ensure that they get enough protein from other sources. Appropriate supplements should be added as well.

BEST MEAT: wild game or 100 percent grass-fed, local lean meats.

SECOND BEST MEAT: organic, naturally raised and hormone and antibiotic free (locally grown when possible).

THIRD BEST MEAT: conventional meat as lean as possible:

- ❏ Flank Steak
- ❏ Chicken Breast
- ❏ Lean Hamburger (beef, bison, buffalo) and minimally processed sausage
- ❏ Chuck Steak, Turkey (including ground and Top Sirloin Steak minimally processed sausage)
- ❏ Veal, Game Hen Breasts
- ❏ Game Meat, Pork Loin, Pork Chops
- ❏ Beef Jerky (low sodium, least amount of ingredients, no soy sauce, ideally organic)

Fish

BEST FISH: wild, fresh or frozen at sea is best.

SECOND BEST FISH: canned fish in water or olive or fish oil, with minimal salt.

- ❏ Bass, Herring, Salmon, Bluefish, Lobster
- ❏ Scallops, Cod, Mackerel, Shrimp, Clams
- ❏ Mahimahi, Tilapia, Crab, Mussels, Trout
- ❏ Crayfish, Orange Roughey, Tuna, Flatfish
- ❏ Oysters, Walleye, Grouper, Perch
- ❏ Haddock, Red Snapper, Halibut, Rockfish

Eggs

BEST EGGS: 100 percent free range, organic.

SECOND BEST EGGS: omega-3 enriched, DHA.

THIRD BEST EGGS: hormone and antibiotic free.

Vegetables

Vegetables should be the main source of carbohydrates. Vegetables are also a good source of protein. Nonstarchy vegetables should be a big part of each meal. Virtually all vegetables offer excellent nutritional value.

BEST VEGETABLES: organic, locally grown, in season; fresh or fresh frozen.

SECOND BEST VEGETABLES: nonorganic, locally grown; fresh or fresh frozen.

THIRD BEST VEGETABLES: bought fresh at the store, either grown as locally as possible or imported organic.

- ❏ Artichoke, Celery, Mushrooms, Seaweed
- ❏ Asparagus, Collards, Mustard Greens, Beets, Cucumber, Onions, Spinach
- ❏ Beet Greens, Dandelion, Parsnip, Swiss Chard
- ❏ Bell Peppers, Eggplant, Parsley, Sweet Potato/Yam
- ❏ Broccoli, Endive, Peppers (all kinds), Tomato
- ❏ Brussels Sprouts, Green Onions, Pumpkin, Tomatillos
- ❏ Cabbage, Kale, Purslane, Turnip Greens

- ❏ Carrots, Kohlrabi, Radish, Turnips
- ❏ Cauliflower, Lettuce, Rutabaga, Watercress

Fruits

BEST FRUIT SOURCE: organic, locally grown, in season; fresh or fresh frozen.

SECOND BEST FRUIT SOURCE: nonorganic, locally grown; fresh or fresh frozen.

THIRD BEST FRUIT SOURCE: bought fresh at the store, either grown as locally as possible or imported organic.

- ❏ Apple, Cherries, Lychee, Plums
- ❏ Apricot, Cranberries, Mango, Pomegranate
- ❏ Avocado, Dates, Nectarine, Raspberries
- ❏ Banana, Figs, Orange, Rhubarb
- ❏ Blackberries, Gooseberries, Passion Fruit, Strawberries
- ❏ Blueberries, Grapes, Papaya, Star Fruit
- ❏ Boysenberries, Honeydew Melon, Peaches, Tangerine
- ❏ Cantaloupe, Kiwi, Pears, Watermelon
- ❏ Cassava Melon, Lemon, Persimmon
- ❏ Cherimoya, Lime, Pineapple
- ❏ Dried Fruit (unsweetened, unsulfured, and limit the quantity)

Nuts and Seeds

Nuts and seeds pack protein, fatty acids, enzymes, antioxidants, as well as vitamins and minerals (especially potassium and magnesium). Nuts in moderation are healthy, but overconsumption will stall weight loss. Cashews are especially delicious but surprisingly high in carbohydrates and also contain a large amount of omega-6 fatty acids (omega-6 fatty acids are less desirable than the omega-3 fatty acids found in fish).

BEST NUTS AND SEEDS: organic, raw, unsalted, and shelled.

SECOND BEST NUTS AND SEEDS: nonorganic, raw, unsalted, and shelled.

- ❏ Almonds, Pecans, Brazil Nuts, Pine Nuts
- ❏ Cashews, Pistachios, Chestnuts, Pumpkin Seeds
- ❏ Hazelnuts, Sesame Seeds, Macadamia Nuts, Sunflower Seeds

OTHER

- ❏ Coconut (raw unsweetened flakes, milk)
- ❏ Almond Milk (organic with minimal ingredients)
- ❏ Nut Flours (minimize use)
- ❏ Nut/Seed Butters (no peanut butter)

Fats

Fat is essential to your well-being and happiness. Certain types of fat provide a great source of energy and are an essential part of many cellular and hormonal processes. Fat makes people feel full.

OILS: a good source of fat.

BEST OILS: organic extra-virgin oils packed in dark bottles.

SECOND BEST OILS: nonorganic extra-virgin oils packed in dark bottles.

THIRD BEST OILS: organic virgin or nonorganic virgin all in dark bottles.

- ❏ **Avocado (on the fruit list but considered a fat source more than a fruit)**
- ❏ Olive Oil, Walnut Oil
- ❏ Canola Oils, Flaxseed, Coconut Oil

Herbs, Spices, and Anything Nice

Avoid excessive amounts of sugar and salt.

- ❏ Allspice, Ginseng, Pepper
- ❏ Anise, Green Tea, Peppermint
- ❏ Basil, Horseradish, Poppy Seed
- ❏ Bay Leaf, Jalapeño Peppers, Pomegranate Seeds
- ❏ Cardamon, Jasmine, Rosemary
- ❏ Cayenne Pepper, Lavender, Safflower
- ❏ Celery Seed, Lemon Balm, Saffron
- ❏ Chamomile, Lemon Basil, Sage
- ❏ Chili, Lemon Mint, Sea Salt*
- ❏ Chives, Lemon Myrtle, Spearmint

- ❑ Cilantro/Coriander, Lemon Thyme
- ❑ Cloves, Licorice, Tamarind
- ❑ Cumin, Majoram, Tarragon
- ❑ Curry Leaves, Mint, Tea
- ❑ Cocoa, Mustard Seed, Thai Basil
- ❑ Dandelion, Myrtle, Thyme
- ❑ Dill, Nutmeg, Turmeric
- ❑ Fenugreek, Oregano, Vanilla
- ❑ Ginger, Paprika, Wasabi
- ❑ Ginkgo, Parsley, Wattleseed

OTHER

- ❑ Raw Apple Cider Vinegar (avoid all other vinegars—they may be made from grain and therefore are not grain or gluten free—use lime or lemon juice as a substitute for vinegar)
- ❑ Honey (raw, organic locally grown honey is preferable; honey is still a form of sugar, so use very minimally or avoid completely)
- ❑ Agave Nectar (raw, organic locally grown agave is preferable; agave is still a form of sugar, so use very minimally or avoid completely; honey is actually better for you than agave)

Beverages

- ❑ Clean Filtered Water, Coffee (try to limit)
- ❑ Herbal Tea, Black or Green Tea

*Use in moderation—try to avoid.

Substitution, Scaling, and Standards

If we did all the things we are capable of, we would literally astound ourselves.
—THOMAS EDISON

A wide variety of equipment is required for SEALFIT. Many of the exercises prescribed are initially difficult to execute. Please don't get discouraged. Remember what I said at the beginning of SEALFIT–Navy SEAL training started with a single push-up. You can do this! Let's talk about substitution and scaling. Substitution occurs when you substitute one exercise for another because:

- You don't have the right equipment.
- Your body isn't working the way you're asking it to.
- You don't have a partner for the "partner workout."
- You have a legitimate injury that you need to work around.

It's impossible to account for every situation. I suggest that you join a coached training environment like a CrossFit gym or hire a private trainer (hopefully both will have the expertise to guide you, but there's no guarantee). SEALFIT is here to help, so please feel free to call us at (760) 634-1833.

Substitutions

- **ROWER:** SDHP at 75#/55# for the same relative duration as the row.

- **BUDDY CARRY OR PULL:** Buddy Carry—farmer's carry at body weight for 400m. Pull—sprints with medicine ball, although this doesn't equate to the intensity of a buddy pull. Can you find a better substitute with your available tools?

- **GHD:** wall ball sit-ups or kettlebell sit-ups starting with the kettlebell overhead. Sit up holding the kettlebell and hold it in front of you.

- **ROPE-TOWEL PULL-UPS (SIX PER ROPE ASCENT):** If you can't climb the rope, hold it and lower yourself to the ground. Maintain a straight back and tight core—an inverted plank position. Form is crucial for the climb—use your feet to hold you by standing on the rope, one foot on top of the other. Use your arms only to reach higher for the next handhold.

- **NO SANDBAG?** Make one.

- **NO WEIGHT VEST?** Buy one, or carry a day pack with 20 pounds wrapped in a blanket.

- **NO KETTLEBELL?** Use a dumbbell.

- **NO BARBELL OR PULL-UP BARS?** *Hmmm*—you'll need to buy both or find an Olympic lifting gym that has a good pull-up station. Globo Gyms are not the answer. Many SEALFIT athletes have been kicked out of Globo Gyms because they scare the people "working out"! CrossFit gyms are popping up all across America—find one and tell them you're training for SEALFIT. You will probably find like-minded SEALFIT trainees to build a team.

Scaling

- **PULL-UPS:** Jumping and band-assisted pull-ups will train you to perform a dead hang and a kip. Kipping pull-ups are a great skill to learn. I don't have the ability to teach those through print at this time. Come to SEALFIT HQ and we'll teach you the kip and butterfly pull-up.

- **PUSH-UPS:** Use your knees, or a GHD to push against. For handstand push-ups (HSPU), elevate your feet on a box and execute inverted push-ups, or use two bands from a pull-up bar. Put one hand over the bar, the other hand through the band, and place your head through the second band. Wrap it around your shoulders so it supports you as you perform the HSPU directly under the pull-up bar. This is effective, but slightly scary on the kick-up. Just do it!

- **WEIGHTED MOVEMENTS:** Scale the load until you can handle it. A good coach is worth his weight in iron for support in learning the lifts properly. We teach them all at SEALFIT Academy.

- **OTHER SCALING ISSUES:** Please see our Web site or give us a call at (760) 634-1833.

Strength Standards

SEALFIT standards establish loads during maximal rep (i.e., 1 RM, 3 RM) sessions. This is a simple and clean way to measure relative strength, a crucial aspect of getting SEALFIT. Strength builds a foundation of performance and confidence. Combined with good flexibility, joint mobility, and core stability, it enhances your durability as both an athlete and professional.

STRENGTH STANDARDS (RELATIVE TO BODY WEIGHT)

BACK SQUAT:	Men 1.5 BW	Women 1.0 BW
DEADLIFT:	Men 2.0 BW	Women 1.5 BW
PUSH PRESS:	Men 1.0 BW	Women .75 BW
BENCH PRESS:	Men 1.5 BW	Women 1.0 BW
SQUAT CLEAN:	Men 1.25 BW	Women 1.0 BW
CLEAN AND JERK:	Men 1.0 BW	Women .75 BW

Stamina Standards

Stamina allows you to move your body more efficiently and to carry heavy loads further.

BODY-WEIGHT MOVEMENT STANDARDS (ELITE LEVEL)

BW SQUAT: > 100 in 2 minutes

BW PUSH-UP: > 100 in 2 minutes

BW PULL-UP: > 20 in 2 minutes

BW SIT-UP: > 100 in 2 minutes

Endurance Standards

Run: 1.5 miles in 9:00

Run: 3 miles in 20:00

Run: 6 miles in 45:00

Run: 14 miles until completion

Ruck: 26 miles with 40# until completion

Swim: 500 meters in 8:00

Swim: 1 mile in 35:00

Row: 2,000 meters in 7:45

Row: 5,000 meters in 20:00

Running and Rucking Form

Your running form makes a big difference in terms of increasing efficiency, increasing speed, and decreasing joint impact. We endorse *pose* running for LSD efforts. Key points:

- "Fall forward" into the next step.
- Stand tall and don't run hunched over.
- Land flat on the mid to forward part of the foot (rather than the traditional heel-toe strike).
- Take shorter steps for a faster repetition cadence (90 steps per minute).
- Move foot in circular rotation.
- Swing arm forward.

Rucking is a great training tool, but can put serious strain on your body. Try to limit it to a couple of times per month. Guidelines:

- Don't jog or run with your pack. Rather, step up your walking pace. If you want to run with load use a weight vest (i.e., with Murph).
- Land flat footed.
- Lean into the stride—strive to "fall to" the next step, similar to pose running.
- Increase your cadence by taking smaller and faster steps.

- Break in your boots.

- Wear chafing gear and two pairs of socks.

- Prepare your feet for a long ruck hike with 2nd Skin or moleskin to prevent blisters. Treat blisters immediately.

- Carry the load on your hips, not your shoulders. Hip belts were invented for this, so use them.

Definitions, Acronyms, and Abbreviations

FUNCTIONAL STRENGTH: To get strong in a functional manner—such as squatting, lifting, pushing, and pulling—we use movements that are natural, safe, and holistic. Engage the core before using the extremities. Functional strength development requires simultaneous core strength development. SEALFIT combines strength work and durability to ensure core stability grows alongside strength.

RELATIVE STRENGTH: Strength exhibited is relative to the size of the delivery vehicle. A 165-pound man with a 300-pound deadlift (1.8 pounds lifted per pound of body weight) is relatively stronger than a 210-pound man with a 350-pound deadlift (1.6) even though the larger man is lifting more weight.

ABSOLUTE STRENGTH: Defined as the amount of musculoskeletal force one can generate for an all-out effort, irrespective of time or body weight.

This form of strength can be demonstrated or tested in the weight room during the performance of a maximal, single-repetition lift. While only powerlifters, Olympic lifters, and CrossFitters will need to demonstrate this type of strength in competition, all athletes need to develop absolute strength as a foundation for other biomotor abilities such as strength speed, strength endurance, agility, etc.

Absolute strength is displayed through two muscular actions:

CONCENTRIC MOVEMENT: The ability to overcome a resistance through muscular contraction. The muscle shortens as it develops tension.

ECCENTRIC MOVEMENT: Displayed when a muscle lengthens as it yields to a resistance. Eccentric strength is normally 30–50 percent greater than concentric strength, meaning that you can lower significantly more weight in good control than you can actually lift.

OLYMPIC LIFTS: Advanced movements that teach the ability to apply force in the proper sequence—from the core to the extremities. Olympic lifts also develop the ability to apply strength, speed, and power to accelerate an object from a dead stand, which can translate to a valuable skill in a fight or a crisis. The lifts teach one to receive force from a moving body (i.e., catching the load at the bottom of the snatch or the top of the clean). The only downside to Olympic lifts is that they are highly technical skills that take many moons to develop. As with all things in SEALFIT, patience is a virtue.

PRIMARY AND SUPPLEMENTAL STRENGTH EXERCISES: As discussed earlier, SEALFIT's primary exercises for strength include the back squat, push press, deadlift, and bench press. These lifts were chosen for a reason, but they're not the only lifts we use. We rely on the Olympic lifts, complexes, kettlebells, dumbbells, sandbags, tires, sledgehammers, logs, and a variety of body weight exercises. We never run out of fun toys to play with.

SUPPLEMENTAL STRENGTH EXERCISES: Supplemental strength exercises are used in work capacity training and on occasion in lieu of a primary strength. These include but are not limited to:

TOTAL BODY

- Olympic lifts
- complexes—barbell complex, Curtis P, Frog Complex, Man Maker
- thruster
- tire flips and sledge strikes
- sandbag get-ups and drills
- Turkish get-ups
- kettlebell and dumbbell work

UPPER BODY

- push-up variations
- pull-up variations
- ring dips, push-ups, and muscle-ups
- handstand push-ups
- buddy carry
- farmer's carry, farmer's walk
- other team drills

LOWER BODY

- lunge variations
- step-ups
- air squats
- buddy pulls with bands

Acronyms and Abbreviations

AMRAP: as many rounds or reps as possible

ATG: ass to grass

BBPlex: barbell complex

BP: bench press

BS: back squat

BW: body weight

CLN: clean

C&J: clean and jerk

C2: Concept II rowing machine

DL: deadlift

DB: dumbbell

FS: front squat

GHD back or hip extension: glute-ham raise (developer); posterior chain exercise, like a back extension

GHD sit-up: sit-up done on the glute-ham developer bench

GPP: general physical preparedness, aka "fitness"

GTG: grease the groove, a protocol of doing many submaximal sets of an exercise throughout the day

HSPU: handstand push-up. Kick up into a handstand (use a wall for balance, if needed), bend arms until nose touches floor, and push back up.

HSQ: hang squat (clean or snatch). Start with bar "at the hang," about knee height. Initiate pull. As the bar rises, drop into a full squat and catch the bar in the racked position. From there, rise to a standing position.

IF: intermittent fasting

KB: kettlebell

KTE: knees to elbows; similar to TTB described below

MetCon: metabolic conditioning workout

MP: military press

MU: muscle-ups. Hanging from rings you do a combination pull-up and dip so you end in an upright support.

OHS: overhead squat—full-depth squat performed while arms are locked out in a wide grip press position above (and usually behind) the head

PC: power clean

Pd: pood, weight measure for kettlebells (we use pounds at SEALFIT)

PR: personal record

PP: push press

PSN: power snatch

PT: physical training

PU: pull-ups, possibly push-ups, depending on the context

Rep: repetition—1 performance of an exercise

RFT: rounds for time

RM: repetition maximum. Your 1 RM is your max lift for 1 rep; your 10 RM is the most you can lift 10 times

ROM: range of motion

Rx'd; as Rx'd: as prescribed; as written—WOD done without any adjustments

SBGU: sandbag get-up (like Turkish get-up, but with sandbag)

SDHP: sumo deadlift high pull

Set: a number of repetitions (i.e., 3 sets of 10 reps, often seen as 3x 10, means do 10 reps, rest, repeat, rest, repeat)

SOP: standard operating procedure

SPP: specific physical preparedness, aka skill training

SN: snatch

SQ: squat

SS: *Starting Strength*; Mark Rippetoe's great book on strength training basics

Subbed: substituted. The CORRECT use of "subbed," as in "substituted," is "I subbed an exercise I can do for one I can't." For example, if you can't do an HSPU, you subbed regular push-ups.

TGU: Turkish get-up

TLU: total, lower, upper

TTB: toes to bar. Hang from the bar, bending only at the waist. Raise your toes to touch the bar, then slowly lower them and repeat.

WO or W/O: workout

WOD: workout of the day

WU: warm-up

ABOUT THE AUTHOR

Mark Divine is the founder of NavySEALs.com, SEALFIT, U.S. Tactical, and Unbeatable Mind. He is also the author of *The Way of the SEAL*, published by Reader's Digest, and *Unbeatable Mind*, which he self-published. Mark started his athletic career as a collegiate swimmer and rower, then became a competitive triathlete and martial artist before attending Officer Candidate School for the Navy in 1989. Mark graduated as Honor Man of his SEAL training class #170 in 1990 and served on active duty for 9 years and in the reserve force for 11. He retired as a commander from the Navy in 2011 after 20 years of total service in the SEAL Teams.

Commander Divine has trained and mentored thousands of Navy SEAL and other Special Operations Forces candidates to succeed in the most demanding military training programs in the world. His success rate with SEALFIT in preparing candidates is unrivaled.

Mark's insights into elite fitness, elite teams, leadership, mental toughness, and warrior spirit development were developed over his 20 years as a SEAL and business leader, 25 years as a martial artist, and 15 years as a yoga practitioner.

Are you ready to EMBRACE THE SUCK again?

If so, then please come join the SEALFIT ONLINE TRAINING PROGRAM & COMMUNITY.

The *8 Weeks to SEALFIT* book was intended to give you a strong foundation to the SEALFIT training program. To continue on your journey, join the SEALFIT Online Training Program & Community of committed athletes and warriors. This is possibly the toughest fitness and mental toughness regimen available in an online format. Coach Divine will push you beyond your threshold with monthly SEALFIT workouts and you will have the added benefit of online journaling, a community of peers, quick connections with other SEALFIT coaches, and all the support and feedback you will need on your personal journey to achieving your goals.

Visit www.SEALFIT.com/8weeks to join today!

As a book owner, you will receive the first 30 days for FREE!

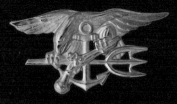
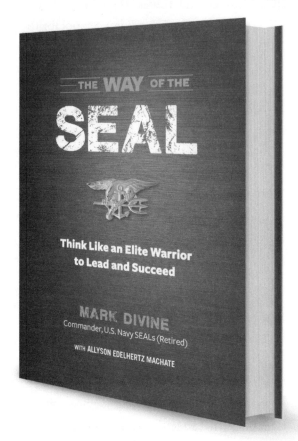